Reducing Global Road Traffic Tragedies

The Lost History of Success in the Rich World Now Urgently Needed in Developing Nations

Reducing Global Road Traffic Tragedies

The Lost History of Success in the Rich World Now Urgently Needed in Developing Nations

Gerald Balcar and Bo Elfving

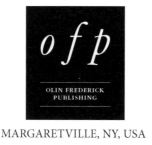

MARGARETVILLE, NY, USA

Copyright © 2016 by Gerald Balcar and Bo Elfving

All rights reserved. No part of this book may be reproduced or transmitted in any form or by any means, electronic or mechanical (including photocopying, recording, or information storage and retrieval) without prior permission from the publisher, except in the case of brief quotations embodied in articles or reviews. For information address Olin Frederick Publishing, Inc., PO Box 200, Margaretville, NY 12455, USA.

Published by Olin Frederick Publishing, Inc,
PO Box 200, Margaretville, NY 12455, USA
Telephone: +1-845-243-3219
Email: info@olinfrederick.com
www.olinfrederick.com

All registered trademarks in this book are property of their respective owners.

Library of Congress Control Number: 2016908134

Balcar, Gerald and Elfving, Bo
Reducing Global Road Traffic Tragedies: The Lost History of Success in the Rich World Now Urgently Needed in Developing Nations / Gerald Balcar and Bo Elfving. – 1st U.S. Edition

p. cm.

Includes bibliographical references and index

ISBN: 978-1-932873-04-7 (paperback)
ISBN: 978-1-932873-05-4 (eBook)

Notice: The information in this book is true and complete to the best of our knowledge. It is offered without guarantee on the part of the authors or Olin Frederick Publishing, Inc. The authors and Olin Frederick Publishing, Inc. disclaim all liability in connection with the use of this book. CS3.

Cover photograph © Brett Cole
Cover background photograph © molotok743/Adobe Stock
Back cover background photograph © ellisia/Adobe Stock

Design by Clas Lindman

For those who seek the truths about reducing road traffic tragedies

Contents

Preface _____ *1*

Introduction _____ *5*
Completing the Quest for Road Safety _____ *7*

Chapter 1 – The Early History of Road Marking _____ *11*
The Development of Funding and Early Traffic Standards _____ *13*
Action for Uniformity _____ *16*

Chapter 2 – Classic Road Marking Tests _____ *19*
Edge Line Tests in Germany _____ *19*
    Bavaria, Lower Saxony and Hesse 1952: Unmarked Roads are Marked ___ *19*
Edge Line Tests in America _____ *20*
    Arizona 1954 _____ *20*
    Utah 1955 _____ *21*
    Michigan 1956 _____ *22*
    Illinois 1956 _____ *22*
    Ohio 1956 _____ *22*
    Kansas 1958 _____ *23*
    Test Conclusions _____ *25*

Chapter 3 – The American Story _____ *27*
Influences in the 1960s _____ *29*
The Highway Safety Act of 1966 _____ *31*
The National Traffic and Motor Vehicle Safety Act of 1966 _____ *33*
The Highway Safety Act of 1973 _____ *34*
The West Milford, NJ Tests _____ *36*
Highlights from The Highway Safety Act of 1973 _____ *42*
The Road Safety Results _____ *45*
A Biographical Note for the American Story _____ *48*

Chapter 4 – The Western European Story _____ *51*
Adopting Road Safety Engineering _____ *52*
Western European Advances in Pavement Marking _____ *54*
Successes in Discouraging Drinking and Driving _____ *56*
Seatbelt Use Laws and Campaigns _____ *58*
Driver Licensing _____ *60*
The Lower Western European Fatality Rates _____ *61*
Vision Zero _____ *64*

Chapter 5 – Advances in Thinking about Road Marking — 65
The Concept of Driver's Vision — 65
Testing of Edge Lines as an Alcohol-Related Crash Countermeasure — 68
The European Commission – COST 331 — 79
The Use of Wider Markings — 82
Report on the Pavement Marking Demonstration Program — 86
The Institute of Transport Economics — 86

Chapter 6 – Road Marking Operations and Priorities — 89
Marking Equipment and Materials — 90
Raised Pavement Markers and Wet Weather — 94
Pavement Marking Operations — 97
Renewal of Pavement Markings — 99
Developing Road Marking Standards — 101
Pedestrians and Cyclists — 104
Budgeting and Priorities — 107

Chapter 7 – Perspectives on Road Traffic Safety — 109
The Elements of Traffic Safety — 110
Advancements in Traffic Safety Thinking — 111
Follow-on Actions to Road Safety Engineering — 114
The Highway Safety Establishment View — 116
Lessons Encountered and Winning Public Support — 121

Chapter 8 – The Story in Low- and Middle-Income Countries — 125
The United Nations' Efforts — 129
The UN/WHO Failings — 137
Recommended Priorities for Low- and Middle-Income Countries — 139
The Role of the Rich World — 144

Conclusion — 147
Getting to Road Traffic Fatality Reductions — 149

Authors' Note — 153
Vehicle Safety Standards and Technology Advancements — 153
Academic Theories and Potential Countermeasures — 154
Global Road Traffic Fatality Data — 154
Acknowledgements — 155

Notes — 157

Glossary — 165

Index — 171

About the Authors — 179

Preface

There is no question that I should have written this book 25 years ago when results of road traffic fatality reduction efforts in the rich world became apparent. By 1990, the average fatality rate per 100,000 population in 23 OECD nations had been reduced from the peak in 1972 of 23.4 to 15.4, a reduction by more than a third. This book tells the story of how this was accomplished. The average rate of those 23 nations has since continually been reduced and was only 5.2 by 2012.

The situation in much of the developing world, however, is the opposite with increasing road traffic crashes, injuries and fatalities. Indeed, the current, inadequate and ineffective efforts led by the United Nations and the World Health Organization aimed at stemming the road traffic tragedy playing out on roads in developing countries are the reasons this book is necessary now in 2016.

As it was, I was involved at the center of a momentous shift in road safety thinking that started essentially in 1971. This shift changed the focus from trying to alter driver and pedestrian behavior and to improve vehicle safety standards to a focus of first improving the safety of existing roads. The leadership and staff of the US House of Representatives Committee on Public Works had lost patience with previous efforts to halt increases in road traffic fatalities. A prior "grand design" highway safety act from the committee in 1966, with a "balanced approach" recommended by the road safety community of the epoch, had not produced the desired results. A companion 1966 act, originating from the US Senate Commerce Committee focused on vehicle safety standards that would eventually make a material contribution, had not yet been effective. New data from the Federal Highway Administration showed widely varying numbers of crashes and deaths on different types of roads. That provided the clue that existing roads could be made safer.

The House Committee invited all with experience in making roads safer to contribute ideas. Representatives from private industry provided concepts not necessarily offered by the traditional road safety community. My first assignment was to prepare a report that fully presented the crash reduction effectiveness, costs and technology of pavement markings, specifically that of reflectorized center lines and edge lines. This was later expanded to include designing and overseeing new pavement marking tests, proving the effectiveness of the markings in reducing road traffic crashes. There were many meetings, formal and informal presentations and testimonies on multiple occasions on both sides of Capitol Hill. I was not a congressman or a staff member, but I was deeply engaged. What developed was a new, science-based philosophy that helped keep a significant share of driver mistakes from happening or from becoming crashes. It came to be called road safety engineering and it worked. This concept was incorporated into American road safety legislation in 1973, and its programs for action were quickly followed in Western Europe. My work on this issue on Capitol Hill lasted more than ten years as the reauthorizations and reevaluations of the 1973 act progressed into the 1980s. During that time, I also participated in related meetings in Europe and Japan.

The main program called for the installation of reflectorized center lines and edge lines on mostly rural, two-lane roads that did not previously have such pavement markings. Most residents today in a rich-world country do not even consider the need for pavement markings. They are already installed everywhere and have been maintained for more than a generation. They are so common and prevalent they are unnoticed. However, many people in low- and middle-income countries have never seen them. Others in those countries see them only in cities or on expressways. Somehow, in recommending programs and actions for low- and middle-income countries, the United Nations and the World Health Organization have largely failed to recognize the need to first focus on making existing roads safer.

Had this book appeared in 1990, it is possible to assume that the UN/WHO might have understood what really produced the fatality reduction results in the rich world. If they had designed an appropriate program focused on the developing world in 2004, or even before, hundreds of thousands of road traffic fatalities and millions of injuries in developing nations might have been averted. The approach taken by the UN/WHO to address this problem is clearly not working. With the recently announced goal to halve the number of global deaths and injuries from road traffic crashes by 2020 as part of the 2030 Agenda for Sustainable Development, a new approach is needed. This book includes recommendations of what to do.

Even though much of this book is based on my personal experience and historical reminiscences, co-author Bo Elfving's voice prevails throughout. This is particularly so in sections discussing recent developments, the present day situation and in the recommendations going forward. His contributions have been essential in making this project a success.

Gerry Balcar
Margaretville, New York
May 18, 2016

Introduction

Road traffic crashes are killing and maiming more people today than ever before. By 2013, annual global road traffic fatalities were estimated to have reached 1.25 million.[1] Of these, 90%, 1.125 million, occurred in low- and middle-income countries.[2] Even though high-income nations had 46% of registered vehicles globally, they only had about 125,000 fatalities, or 10%, of the total.[3] In the 40 years after 1972, road traffic fatalities in 23 high-income OECD countries decreased by 63% with effective crash and death reduction efforts.[4] At the same time, economic growth in low- and middle-income countries saw more households achieve mobility with cars, motorcycles or mopeds, leading to increasing road tragedy.

Never before has there been traffic carnage of this magnitude. Further to the deaths each year in low- and middle-income nations are an estimated 28,000,000 injuries resulting in a probable 1,400,000 permanently disabled people.[5] The economic losses are huge and compound every year. Developing nations pay an annual economic toll for injuries from road traffic crashes of about US $625 billion directly from family, business or public funds that otherwise could be used for economic development.[6]

These losses of death and injury can be significantly reduced, as they have been in the rich world. The road traffic death rate per 100,000 population, often called the population fatality or death rate, in the ten low- and middle-income nations with the largest number of fatalities in 2013 averages 22.7. China's rate is 18.8, India 16.6, Brazil 23.4, Indonesia 15.3, Nigeria 20.5, Pakistan 14.2, Iran 32.1, Thailand 36.2, Ethiopia 25.3, and Viet Nam 24.5.[7]

At the peak of road traffic deaths in high-income countries in 1972, the population fatality rates were similar. The United States had a rate of 26.1; Austria 40.2; France, 35.2; Canada, 28.0; Germany, 27.0; Italy, 22.1; Japan, 19.3; Sweden, 14.7 and the United

Kingdom 14.5.[8] Despite large and expensive efforts to improve driver behavior, annual increases in road traffic deaths persisted. A ground shift in road traffic safety thinking and action began.

The new focus on the safety of existing roads was largely based on field tests of the crash reduction effectiveness of pavement marking undertaken in the 1950s. When reflectorized center lines and edge lines were added to unmarked, mostly rural arterial and collector roads, crashes were reduced by as much as 25% and fatalities as much as 55% (see Chapter 2). Leading theoreticians of traffic safety at the time ignored these findings, however, believing that modifying driver behavior was the main, if not only, way to reduce crashes. Road-building contractors also ignored these findings and espoused that rebuilding roads was necessary for greater road safety. In the United States, these proponents of traditional actions were later overruled at the highest level of government. A new doctrine emerged to make existing roads as safe as possible with road safety improvements. Installing reflectorized center lines with passing zones and edge lines, upgrading intersections, removing obstacles and upgrading rail crossings became the definitive actions of road safety engineering.

Within a few years, a decade of unprecedented increases in road traffic deaths in the United States and Western Europe were reversed. Then, building on that base of declining traffic tragedy resulting from the road safety improvements in the 1970s and 1980s, successful campaigns to discourage drinking and driving and to encourage buckling seatbelts followed. These activities took 30 years. Other campaigns were included, especially in Western Europe, where the average population fatality rate is now only about five. The United States has a current rate of 10.6, Canada is at 6.0 and Japan at 4.7. A few countries have even dipped below 3.[9] Based on the success of these efforts in high-income nations, it is reasonable to conclude that road traffic deaths and injuries in low- and middle-income nations can also be cut substantially. But road safety engineering for these countries is not being promoted, nor is it being deployed, as a primary countermeasure.

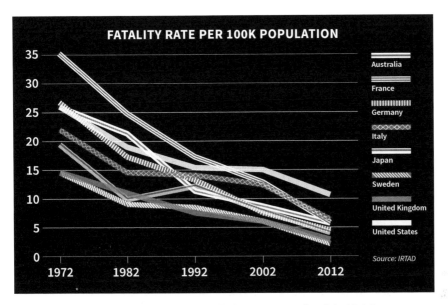

Figure I.1.[10] *Fatality rate per 100,000 population 1972-2012 for eight high-income countries.*

It seems that the knowledge of what happened in the rich world to make existing roads safer was somehow forgotten or marginalized. At the time, there was little real academic work in road safety. It was ten years after the beginning of road safety engineering before the results were known. Road safety engineering actions were implemented and the improvements were kept up, but reports of these achievements did not get noticed or were not written. No government agency or other organization involved held press conferences to explain what happened.

Completing the Quest for Road Safety

The first purpose of this book is to reclaim the little-known history of road safety improvements, the results of road safety engineering. Policy makers at all levels need to know this background, as do highway department managers, operators and engineers. So do journalists, editors and academics, as well as public opinion makers. Road safety engineering is not a panacea for road traffic safety, but is part of a critical and necessary early step.

The second purpose of this book is to make clear to those attempting to reduce road traffic crashes, injuries and deaths in the developing world that the main priority after arranging traffic laws and enforcement should be to move forward with road safety engineering. Raising the safety standards of existing roads saves lives and prevents injuries as soon as the improvements are made. Reflectorized center lines with passing zones and edge lines play a huge role in this. This has been completely missed by those leading the current global crash and death reduction effort.

As world road traffic fatalities increased to over the million-a-year mark, the United Nations stepped visibly forward into the crisis in 2004, assigning the issue to the World Health Organization. Their first action was to produce the 244-page *World Report on Road Traffic Injury Prevention*. Its avowed purpose was "to present a comprehensive overview of what is known about the magnitude, risk factors and impact of road traffic injuries, and about ways to prevent and lessen the impact of road crashes."[11] It was supposed to create discussion. Very little real action ensued. High-income nations, however, had successfully reduced their road traffic crashes, injuries and deaths long before the report was even written. What these nations did was either ignored or misunderstood by the WHO.

A reappraisal began at the UN/WHO. In 2009, a first-ever global ministerial conference on road safety was held in Moscow. Thereafter, a *Global Plan for the Decade of Action for Road Safety 2011-2020* was announced, building on the recommendations of the 2004 report. The proclaimed goal was to save five million lives by 2020.[12] This implied a substantial reduction in the annual tolls of road tragedy in developing countries.

The prevailing excuse for not duplicating what the rich world did seems to be the notion that conditions in developing nations are different. The simple reality is that at its most basic level, the developing world, like the rich world, has rubber-tired vehicles traveling at different speeds on roads. If those roads are made safer, there will be fewer crashes and fewer fatalities. There should be no delay in making the first improvements to existing roads, but an important distinction needs to be made. The WHO Global Plan embraces long-term infrastructure rebuilding, creating or enlarging mass transit services, and expansion of healthcare to care for crash victims. Rebuilding roads will reduce road crashes, increased use of mass transit might reduce the number of vehicles on the roads and better access to healthcare might improve survivability, but these are long-term and separate issues from the immediate need to prevent crashes on existing roads. Road traffic tragedy happening on existing roads and in vehicles already on the roads is the current issue.

Assisting developing nations to build their economies is in the best interest of the rich world. Advancing trade and commerce, and hence furthering economic development, is an acknowledged way to establish and keep democracies sustainable. It now is a task for the rich world to help the developing one with practical traffic safety assistance. The matter in low- and middle-income countries is urgent, but that urgency has not been recognized appropriately by the global road safety community. That traffic tragedy in these countries is largely unabated after twelve years of effort, starting with the WHO 2004 report, borders on scandal. The numbers represent uncountable grief at untimely deaths, of disrupted families and social units, of suffered and treated injuries, and of a build-up of men, women and children with permanent disabilities. All this pain, anguish, frustration, and trauma are in addition to large financial losses.

At the time of our writing (early 2016), no real progress in reducing global road traffic fatalities outside high-income countries has been reported. The rich world needs to push the UN, the WHO and others to step up or to step aside. Current efforts with the current players are not succeeding. If these players cannot dramatically improve what they do and how they do it, it may be necessary for governments of the rich world to take over and reorganize the effort to make it work. Bringing existing road systems in the developing world up to the best possible road safety standards as quickly as possible is essential to begin the process of reducing road traffic crashes, injuries and fatalities.

Roads are a central and critical part of the road traffic safety equation. Crashes happen on roads. The crashes involve humans and vehicles. To prevent crashes, injuries and fatalities, it is necessary to include countermeasures addressing all these three aspects, but with science-based priorities of action. However, it seems as though most road traffic safety discussion heretofore largely ignores the safety condition of existing roads and the need for priorities of action. Priorities of needed actions are recommended in this book. The authors hope you, the reader, will find them compelling.

1
The Early History of Road Marking

A safety-conscious portion of the driving public in the United States has been long involved in traffic operations. The country was not far into the automobile age when calls for the separation of opposite-direction motorized traffic were heard. Apparently, many sensed that the new and faster engine-powered wagons and buggies changed traffic conditions. The speed was no more than 25 km per hour (15 miles per hour) but it was significantly faster and scarier than the six km per hour (four miles per hour) speed of a horse-drawn carriage. Since 1757, speed limits and laws against reckless driving have been established in the United States, but no early law enacted pavement marking.[1] Rather, the popular interest in painted lines on the roads was a presage of things to come.

In 1911, there were hardly more than 640,000 cars and trucks and 349,000 km (217,000 miles) of paved road in the entire country.[2,3] In 2013, there were 267 million registered vehicles and 4.3 million kilometers (2.7 million miles) of paved roads.[4,5] Yet in 1911 there were already 2,000 annual road traffic deaths.[6] That year, a center line was painted along Trenton's River Road in Wayne County, Michigan near Detroit.[7] The work was attributed to Edward N. Hines, the chairman of the Wayne County, Michigan Board of Roads. He said he got the idea after watching a leaky milk wagon leave a white trail along a road.

In 1917, when the number of vehicles in the country had zoomed to over five million and there were 504,000 km (313,000 miles) of paved road (and the number of road traffic deaths had reached over 9,500 annually), the first yellow center line was painted in Multnomah County in Oregon.[8,9,10,11] The idea originated with Multnomah County Sheriff's Deputy Peter Rexford while he rode a bus one rainy night. Rexford justifiably claimed that this was the first yellow center line painted in the country. It was to have significance more than a half century later.

But Multnomah County then became an early doubter of the value of the painted line when it refused to pay for extending such marking. Rexford's boss, Chief Deputy Martin T. Pratt (later elected Sheriff), paid for the added painting out of his own pocket.

Also in 1917, a white center line was hand-painted along "Dead Man's Curve" in Marquette County, Michigan. The then engineer-superintendent of the Marquette County Road Commission, Kenneth Ingalls Sawyer, is credited with directing this work.[12]

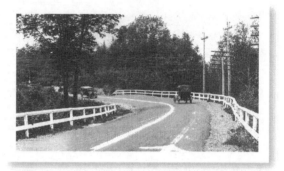

Figure 1.1.[13] *Dead Man's Curve along the Marquette–Negaunee Road in Marquette County, Michigan in 1917.*

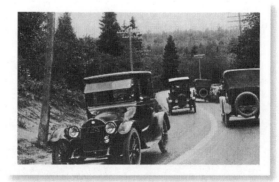

Figure 1.2.[14] *Hand-painted centerline on state highway M-15 (now County Road 492) in Marquette County, Michigan.*

In that same year, 1917, Dr. June McCarroll of Indio, California, suggested that to avoid collisions, white center lines be painted on a main road on which she frequently had to drive. She was turned down by the Riverside County Board of Supervisors. Undaunted, she and some friends then painted the line by hand. But it was not until 1924 that the state of California painted its initial 5,600 km (3,500 miles) of road with a center line. The cost, in 1924 money, was US $163,000 (or $2,228,000 in 2016 dollars).[15]

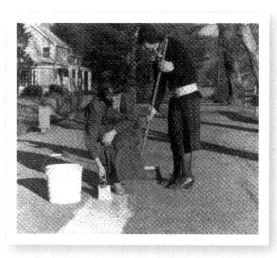

Figure 1.3.[16] *Re-enactment of Dr. June McCarroll painting a center line with a friend.*

These forerunners of modern road delineation were honored, or at least they were intended to be honored. Mr. Hines was inducted posthumously into the Michigan Transportation Hall of Honor. So was Kenneth Ingalls Sawyer. Deputy Rexford was to be celebrated as the originator of the center line. It might have been considered a "first," but later research found that early civilizations had used colored bricks to delineate traffic on their streets. Dr. McCarroll fared best, being memorialized for her contribution to road safety with the dedication of a segment of the Interstate 10 Freeway in Riverside County, California.[17]

The Development of Funding and Early Traffic Standards

Roads marked with center lines were immediately popular with drivers and elicited letters and phone calls to highway departments and newspapers as responses from their start. Drivers liked them, and their demand drove the initial development and installations.

In this case of a new and fundamental traffic control device, it was those most affected, not any government or private organization, who first insisted on the installation and development of the lines. The reaction to the installation of center lines on roads was widespread, telling of the great importance of lines to safe driving from the perspective of the driving public.

The American Association of State Highway Officials (AASHO) was founded in 1914 but it was not until 1927 that it published the first Manual and Specifications for the Manufacture, Display, and Erection of U.S. Standard Road Markers and Signs for rural roads. Of greater importance was the Federal Aid Roads Act of 1916, which opened federal funding for road construction. Others were interested as well. Nine separate auto clubs joined to form the American Automobile Association in 1902. Their first major mission was to call for federal participation in road infrastructure construction. That same year, the American Road Builders Association (ARBA) appeared. The main purpose of this organization was to secure government financing for road construction.

Thus began a long effort in America. Congress passed bills drawing money from general revenues for distribution to the states for road construction from time to time. It was critical for lobbying organizations to keep highway development in front of voters. Then in 1956, with the Interstate Highway System underway, the Highway Trust Fund was established. Initially, a three-cent tax on every gallon of gasoline funded it, rising by 2015 to 18.4 cents per gallon. In 1973 ARBA, having become ARTBA to add transportation builders, objected to funding road safety improvements from the Highway Trust Fund.

In 1930, the National Conference on Street and Highway Safety (NCSHS) produced a Manual on Street Traffic Signs, Signals and Markings for urban roads. This publication mostly dealt with signs and had little coverage about markings, despite the title.

AASHO and NCSHS joined to produce the first *Manual on Uniform Traffic Control Devices* (MUTCD) for the United States in 1935. It was largely advisory, representing the opinions of state highway managers or experts on practices in use across the country. Center lines of white, yellow or black, whichever color would provide the greatest contrast, were allowed, the black being used on white Portland cement concrete roads. Widths of the lines were to be between 10 and 20 cm (4 and 8 inches).

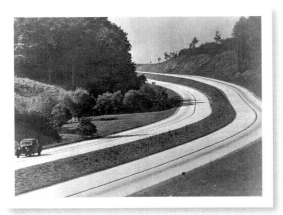

Figure 1.4.[18] *Early, black, center lines on a German Autobahn. These lines did not provide retroreflectivity at night.*

World War II slowed traffic control development, though an interim manual was published in 1942 to address wartime needs. In 1948, a new manual came from the experts. It called for using yellow as a center line color although it allowed lines to be white. Retroreflectorization with glass beads, so lines would retroreflect headlight beams at night, was first tested and used as early as 1937 but was casually treated in the 1948 edition of the manual. It was deemed not to be necessary where street lighting was "adequate." There was a recommendation in the 1948 manual not to install edge lines. This mistake in judgment by the experts of the time began to point to the need for research to define the functions of road markings.

A revision to the manual in 1954 was emphatic on recommending retroreflective road markings. The MUTCD produced in 1961 still allowed white lines as the center line or as a center line with white dashed line passing zones. The dashed line was designated as a 7.5 meter line with a 12 meter gap (25 foot line with a 40 foot gap). The recommended width of the lines was reduced to 10 to 15 cm (4 to 6 inches). This edition of the manual, with the benefit finally of initial crash reduction research, reversed the recommendation against painting edge lines.

Action for Uniformity

The Federal Highway Administration (FHWA) was formed in 1967 to take over the national road-building program of the era under the Department of Transportation. It consolidated functions of the Bureau of Public Roads, which had alternately been part of the Department of Agriculture and the Department of Commerce. When the FHWA assumed authority for the MUTCD in 1971, there were some major changes. Principally, the MUTCD was now a federal government publication. If the word "shall" was used with a requirement, it was now mandatory. In charge of producing the MUTCD was Robert E. Connor of the Office of Traffic Operations. He was effectively the Chief Traffic Engineer of the United States. In 1984, he received the Theodore M. Matson Memorial Award, the highest award given by the Institute of Traffic Engineers.[19] In the award declaration he was referred to as "Mr. Uniformity." He believed the United States should have uniform signs, signals and, most importantly, road markings instead of leaving the matter to individual states. Not everyone initially agreed on uniformity. Some states still thought they had the right and responsibility to mark their roads and erect signs as they saw fit for the best interests of their citizens.

In some states, the division in opinion was even on the county level. That turned into a unique advantage for those seeking uniformity. In 1971, Potters Industries, the American multinational producer of glass beads that were used to retroreflectorize road markings, embarked on a large materials and paint formulation test in West Milford, New Jersey. With excellent cooperation from the township government, a test field of twenty miles of roads was painted. Compared were what was then the generally accepted thickness of paint and measure of beads with alternative formulations. Other important tests included beads made from higher refractive index glasses and thermoplastic and epoxy materials. Bob Connor and FHWA personnel were frequent visitors to observe the testing.

It happened that West Milford was located in Passaic County, New Jersey, which painted its roads with white edge lines and a center line without passing zones indicated. To the west was Sussex County, which also used only white lines but showed passing zones. To the south was Morris County which used the 1961 MUTCD suggestion of yellow center lines with white dashed lines to show passing zones. In addition to these variations, the Potters test used the soon-to-be-proposed all-yellow center lines and dashed lines.

In this area of about 3,000 square km (1,150 square miles) and population of 150,000, drivers were familiar with more than one road marking system. In Washington, DC, resistance to uniformity had coalesced around the only possible claim, namely, that people did not care. The FHWA organized a fully randomized and well-structured survey of West Milford families with cars. Ninety-eight percent favored uniformity; 94% chose the all-yellow center line system. The 1971 MUTCD established national uniformity with the all-yellow center lines.

In Western Europe, the public liking for, and then demand for, pavement markings similarly drove their installation. Most nations chose white-only road markings. The argument was, and continues to be, that white produces greater contrast with road surfaces. Some nations were also using wider lines. From post-World War I through the 1940s, roads got marked because those behind the wheels in Western Europe and North America wanted them center lined.

When edge lines appeared, the combination of center lines and edge lines was even more popular and generated additional positive responses from drivers to highway departments and the media. But obviously they were more expensive to install. Marking a two-lane road with center lines and edge lines would double the cost of installation compared to installing only center lines. Highway department wisdom is that once roads are marked, especially with edge lines, the driving public would demand they remain marked. This caused concern from highway departments as the additional cost would strain their budgets.

During the same period, the traffic control manuals on both

sides of the Atlantic were written, largely by experts. Some theory had evolved, but little research had been conducted. Then, as the 1950s arrived, so did questions: "What are we doing and why are we spending all this money?" The cost of installing center lines and edge lines may have been one factor for pause. Another concern was to determine which roads, and with what traffic counts, should have road markings installed? It was time to get serious about road marking research.

2

Classic Road Marking Tests

By the early 1950s, edge lines had appeared in some jurisdictions and were very popular with drivers. European nations and American states were installing them by public demand. They also cost twice as much as center lines alone. Were they worth it? That question had to be addressed as well as the value of center-line marking. It was hard to predict what the results would be when comparing crash data before and after the installation of road markings on test roads. As it was, the results were more than surprising.

Edge Line Tests in Germany

Bavaria, Lower Saxony and Hesse 1952:
Unmarked Roads are Marked[1]

The first action was in Germany, where recovery from World War II strained budgets as was the case in most of Europe. Two tests on two-lane roads were planned starting in 1952 and were completed in 1958.

On the B-2 (B=Bundesstrasse or Federal Highway) from Munich to Garmisch-Partenkirchen in Bavaria, center lines were added with post delineators that had reflectors in both directions along each side. Average daily traffic on the road ranged from 4,000 to 8,600 vehicles. The length of the test road was 90 km (56 miles).

On the B-3 in Lower Saxony between Hanover and Celle, center lines were added with post delineators but edge lines were also added. The length of the road for this test was 40 km (25 miles). Average daily traffic was reported to range from 5,000 to 6,500 vehicles.

These tests compared crash experience in 1956 before, and in

1957 after, road markings and post delineators were added to the test roads. The researchers in Lower Saxony were aware of the lack of true control segments that would show crash experience on untreated roads. They removed crashes caused by ice, snow, rain and animals from the counts. They also took out those caused by inebriation, which subsequent tests showed might not have been appropriate. The results were nonetheless startling.

On the B-2, total crashes were reported to have been reduced by 10%.

On the B-3, the total crash reduction was 25% with a 47% reduction in injury crashes and a 55% reduction in fatal crashes.

No one expected such a dramatic impact. The researchers in Bavaria concluded that the addition of edge lines to the test in Lower Saxony was responsible for the results. Thinking about road marking in Germany and elsewhere started to change.

Another test was then in order and was conducted in the state of Hesse on the 3004 and 3024 roads from Hohemark (Oberursel) to the Grosser Feldberg park. The distance of this test section was 12 km (8 miles). The test section was treated with center lines, edge lines and post delineators. The years compared were 1958, the before-treatment year with an average daily traffic of 2,194, and 1960, the after-treatment year when the average daily traffic was 2,850. Crashes declined 40% and injuries declined 58%. The findings continued to be astonishing. Painting edge lines on rural roads could evidently reduce crashes, injuries and fatalities. The highway authorities of Western Europe continued marking their roads.

Edge Line Tests in America

Arizona 1954[2]

Major tests were not far off in the United States. In *Traffic Quarterly* in April 1955, William E. Willey, a high ranking engineer in the Arizona Department of Highways, told a remarkable story. It happened in the winter of 1953, at a public traffic safety meeting of the Phoenix Community Council:

"A gentleman in the audience said he believed that many people ran off the shoulder because they didn't know where the shoulder was. He suggested that perhaps a white stripe adjacent to the shoulder on an asphalt highway would identify both the danger area and promote traffic safety. As a member of the panel of so-called experts I made a note of the suggestion."

The suggestion led to two tests with simultaneous controls. 48 km (30 mile) segments of 24 km (15 miles) with edge lines and 24 km (15 miles) of unmarked control segments would be installed on US 89 near Nogales and on US 66 west of Kingman. In the section north of Nogales, 18 crashes occurred during the observation period of three months. Two of these resulted in fatalities, which, with 13 others, occurred in the unmarked control section. Only three happened where edge lines were installed.

On the section near Kingman, 35 crashes occurred during the observation period of 8 months. One of these resulted in a fatality. Eleven were on the fully marked segment. The fatal crash and 23 others were on the unmarked control section.

Once again, there was surprise at the tested effectiveness of edge lines.

Utah 1955[3]

James R. Halverson, then Chief Traffic Engineer of the State Road Commission of Utah, told of other public responses in *Traffic Safety* in September 1957:

"Common sense tells us that [edge lines] are of great help to motorists at night. [This has been] reinforced by newspaper editorials and letters received complimenting the department on the pavement edge markings."

The before and after test in Utah was on 13 km (8 miles) of State Route 48 leading to the Bingham Copper Mine. Crashes were reduced after the installation of edge lines, but the resulting numbers were judged to be too small for statistical analysis. But a concurrent test of lateral position on the roads with and without edge lines resulted in clear behavioral changes by drivers toward the center of the lanes.

Michigan 1956[4]

The test of edge lines by the Michigan Highway Department was on 65 km (40 miles) of Highway 12 between Jonesville and Clinton (Hillsdale and Lenawee Counties). A year of crash experience was recorded before edge lines were installed. The following 12 months were the test period.

Total crashes were reduced 11% from 199 to 177. Fatalities were reduced from five to one. Personal injuries fell from 112 to 60, or by 46%.

Illinois 1956[5]

This was a big test. A total of 615 km (381 miles) of two-lane roads were center-lined but not edge-lined in 1956 which was the before-treatment year. Edge lines were then added in 1957, and 1958 became the after-treatment year. The surfaces tested were Portland cement concrete and blacktop separated into road widths of less than 6 meters and more than 6 meters (20 feet).

Total crashes were reduced from 683 to 540, or by 21%. Injuries were reduced from 561 to 470, or by 16%. Fatalities were reduced from 25 to 15, or by 40%. A clue as to one possible reason for the larger fatality and injury reductions experienced in tests was that head-on collisions were reduced 59%.

The German results seemed to have been repeated. In Illinois, Lower Saxony and Hesse, and in every future test of crash reduction, regardless of venue, the percentages of serious crashes reduced have always been higher than the percentages of reduction in total crashes.

Ohio 1956[6]

The Ohio Department of Highways, under the leadership of traffic engineer John Musick, took a very serious look at edge marking two-lane roads in 1956 and designed a test of simultaneous controls. The test roads would be marked with both center lines and edge lines. Sections of road adjacent to the test roads would be marked with center lines only and then observed and compared with the test sections before and after. The test was designed to absorb variations in weather conditions.

Throughout the state, engineers installed test segments in nine of the twelve highway department districts. These were approximately 20 km (12 mile) long and split evenly between test roads with both center lines and edge lines as well as passing zones, and control sections with only center lines and passing zones. The road widths were not less than 6 meters (20 feet) or more than 7.3 meters (24 feet). Shoulders were a curb to 4 meters (14 feet) wide, but were reported to be mostly 1 to 2.5 meters (4 to 8 feet) wide. Both the test and control sections would be measured before and after and compared for results of crash behavior.

The results lent a good example of the management of such tests with independent control roads. Total crashes increased 28% and injury crashes increased 50% on the control roads. Total crashes increased 2.4% and injury crashes decreased 8.6% on the test roads. The algorithms that match control results with test results take into account traffic and weather events. The researchers calculated a 19% decrease in total crashes and a 37% decrease in injury crashes on the test sections versus the control sections. Night crashes were reduced by 35% and day crashes by 8%.

The design of the controls served their intended purpose. The results proving the effectiveness of edge lines continued to be spectacular.

Kansas 1958[7]

The Kansas Highway Department kept records of the one year before and one year after crash results from early painting of edge lines in 1957 on eight sections of 140 km (88 miles) of rural roads. They reported a 25% reduction in crashes, a 33% decrease in personal injury crashes and a 50% decrease in fatal crashes.

On another 140 km (88 miles) of twelve sections painted with edge lines in 1958, the department recorded a decrease of 19.6% in total crashes, a 22% decrease in injury crashes and a 54.5% decrease in fatal crashes.

In 1959, edge lines were installed on an additional 15 road sections totaling 330 km (204 miles). From these sections treated with edge lines, the department reported a decrease of 11% in total crashes, an increase of 5% in injury crashes and a decrease of 30% in fatal crashes.

These findings were summarized into a three-year before-and-after study. The result was a decrease of 16.5% in total crashes, a 12.6% decrease in personal injury crashes and a 44.4% decrease in fatal crashes.

In 1960, the question of the controls or standards to which test sections were compared again surfaced. Were before and after tests meaningful? In the before period on the same road, weather conditions may have been significantly more severe in the before time producing a surplus of crashes. Or, conversely, weather could have been much better in the year after to generate fewer crashes. The researchers of Lower Saxony took out the weather related crashes to better focus their before and after observations. The test in Ohio showed that control roads should be active simultaneously with the test roads, and located in close proximity, to provide similar conditions, similar drivers and similar vehicles.

The Ohio protocol was adopted for a new test. Kansas sought to improve on it with a study in cooperation with the old federal Bureau of Public Roads. The program located 29 study sections around the state. Each section would be about 20 km (12 miles) long. Half of each section would be edge-lined with center lines and passing zones and half of the section with only center lines and passing zones which would serve as control sections. The criteria were:

- The road width would be between 6 and 8 meters (20 and 26 feet)
- The turf shoulder would be between 30 and 180 cm (1 and 6 feet) wide
- Minimum traffic variations with not less than 1,000 vehicles per day
- Uniform roadside rural culture
- A minimum of one crash per mile per year
- Minimum section length of 16 km (10 miles)

The end result of this test was that no significant conclusions were drawn except that fatalities were reduced in the test segments. Overall, crashes and injuries decreased more on the control roads. Fatalities increased on the control roads, however, and decreased on the test roads. Of all of the tests, this test had the lowest crashes per km (mile) per year, less than half compared to the test and control roads in Ohio, where the same protocol was used.

Test Conclusions

With the exception of the second Kansas test, the other tests had much commonality. The experts of Lower Saxony culled out crashes due to weather, animals and intoxicated drivers and still recorded a 25% reduction in crashes, an over 40% reduction in injury crashes and a 55% reduction in fatal crashes. In every test, the presence of edge lines, and indeed center lines, has been shown to mitigate more severe crashes. Some data suggests that because of the road markings, there were fewer head-on collisions. In these classic tests, it is always clear that injuries and deaths are especially reduced when roads are treated with both edge lines and center lines. This became a regular finding.

Many additional tests of road marking have been conducted and yet more papers about road marking have been written. However, these tests are the classics. The safety effectiveness revealed was remarkable and encouraging to those eager to provide a significant countermeasure to traffic tragedy. Others, those who would have to spend millions of dollars to install road markings in their districts, were in disbelief. Sharing the disbelief were the construction companies and other vendors who regularly bid on the contracts for new or expanded roads. They were encouraged by the inconclusive Kansas test. The traditional hierarchy of road safety likewise was in disbelief and objected. Their message was that increased road safety, and reduced death and injury, could only be realized through changing driver behavior to reduce speeds, to obey the laws and signs and to stop drinking and driving.

The inconclusive Kansas test may have been "the doubt heard round the world." Many in different countries died or were injured because of it. The argument from the construction industry was that there was no way to improve road safety except by building better roads. The contractors or their representatives, resident in all of the decision making offices, cautioned against any expanded installations of center lines and edge lines. Road safety engineering has a natural opponent in the construction industry when it comes to budget discussions in highway departments. The issue is the budget allocation of money that creates or sustains jobs in a city, town, county or state. Few highway departments jumped into expanding road marking. They did what they had to do without upsetting the proponents among the driving public.

It remained for a crisis of increasing road traffic deaths and injuries in the United States to be resolved by a momentous change in road safety thinking. The classic tests played a large role in the decision in the United States for further road marking action, resulting in extensive installation of retroreflective center lines and edge lines on unmarked rural roads. These tests were instrumental in shifting the traffic safety focus from the actions of drivers to the effect of the safety character of the road environment on drivers. What happened in America first was quickly adopted in other high-income nations.

3

The American Story

American drivers were among the first to request, and then demand, road delineation. This occurred as the use of cars, trucks, and busses soared, bringing undreamed of mobility and convenience to middle-class working people. Motorized vehicles also brought economy and convenience to freight and delivery operations. Regrettably, these years also included two world wars. Profound change quickly began following the armistice of 1918, much of it based on this four-wheeled, self-powered technology. Vehicle registrations, vehicle miles traveled, and road traffic injuries and deaths rose rapidly.

The deaths and injuries, and the crash costs of the automobile age, did not go unnoticed in the United States. Immediately after World War II, President Harry Truman began a series of conferences in Washington, DC, in which he personally appeared in order to bring attention to road safety. His objective was to get the individual states to establish laws, licensing procedures, and enforcement practices that were uniform and effective. Further, there were appeals to everyone to obey the traffic laws and to drive safely. Aside from this, much time was spent by states on road construction issues and funding thereof. There were continued discussions about the idea of a national highway system.

The Eisenhower administration continued these traffic safety initiatives. Cities and towns were urged to establish or enhance safety organizations to remind the public of the need for safe driving and safe walking on or around roads. A National Action Committee for Highway Safety was established in 1954. Federal standards for traffic safety were controversial and failed to pass in Congress because of the politically sensitive issue of the federal government infringing on states' rights. The concept of a national highway system also failed for the same reason.

When the Interstate and Defense Highway system was created by the Federal Aid Highway Act of 1956, the means for imposing federal traffic standards were created. The act established the Highway Trust Fund, into which a federal tax of three cents per gallon of gasoline was deposited. This provided from 50% to 90% of funding for the states to construct roads. With the federal funding to the states came federal authority. The urgings for better traffic safety continued.

It was not until the early 1960s, when most families had a car and more than a few had two, that the United States began in earnest to focus on road safety issues. For nearly 30 years prior to 1961, the annual total of road traffic fatalities in the United States, always the figure most watched, had hovered around 35,000. Then in 1962, that total increased by 3,000 and continued to increase annually thereafter. Proportional increases in crashes and injuries also occurred, causing much public media and political attention. The idea of continued, and inescapable, increases in traffic fatalities seemed possible. By 1965, traffic deaths reached 47,000, an increase of 30% compared to 1961.[1] There was further anxiety as the death rate per 100,000 population rose from 19.8 to 24.2 during that same four year period.[2] The matter became a national crisis.

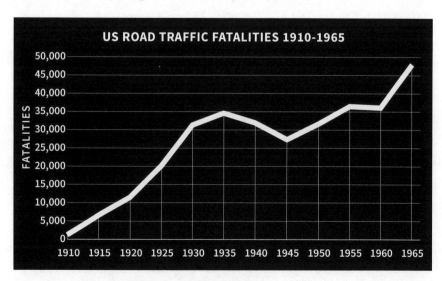

Figure 3.1.[3] *US Road Traffic Fatalities 1910-1965.*

Influences in the 1960s

In the 1960s, a seemingly new way of looking at road safety emerged with Dr. William Haddon, Jr., a graduate of Massachusetts Institute of Technology and Harvard University Medical School. With a degree in Public Health, also from Harvard, he elected not to practice medicine and instead worked for the New York State Department of Public Health for ten years. He was a profuse writer of research and commentary on poisons, body lice, head trauma, routes of infection, pesticides, x-ray usage, skiing accidents and the effect of sports on health. His first published venture in road safety was on alcohol and single-vehicle crashes in 1959. In 1961, he called attention to vehicle design and its effect on road safety. He did some work on driver licensing requirements. In 1962, he produced an analysis of strategies aimed at car safety design.[4]

Haddon was among the first to argue that injury is a disease, that road safety was a public health issue, and suggested a concept of epidemiology to solve it. As diseases are caused by pathological agents, he, and others who agreed with him, suggested that agents like visual defects, stress, alcoholism, and other conditions likewise influenced traffic crashes. Haddon won leadership amongst road safety activists and with that, notoriety. He became a frequent speaker at highway and health conferences and meetings. President Lyndon Johnson chose him as the first head of the National Traffic Safety Agency in October 1966 and while there, he oversaw the issuance of the first government standards for car safety design. In March 1969, he became President of the Insurance Institute for Highway Safety (IIHS) and remained there for the rest of his career. After he left the National Traffic Safety Agency, it became the National Highway Traffic Safety Administration (NHTSA) in 1970.

Haddon is most known for his concept of a nine-part matrix for identifying different variables of road traffic crashes at the different phases of crashes. He later updated it to a twelve-part matrix by splitting the environment factor into separate physical and socio-economic environments. He applied principles of public health to the problem of traffic safety and injury prevention, which was novel and served the purpose of distilling the complexity of the issue. It elicited much comment and gained its own notoriety. Even though the matrix included reference to the road as an element of the physical environment, the critical role of roads in crash prevention went unrecognized. The matrix was a welcome tool for analysis, but it did not provide solutions or priorities of action to meaningfully prevent road traffic crashes. The Haddon Matrix was later modified for use in analyzing issues other than road traffic crashes.

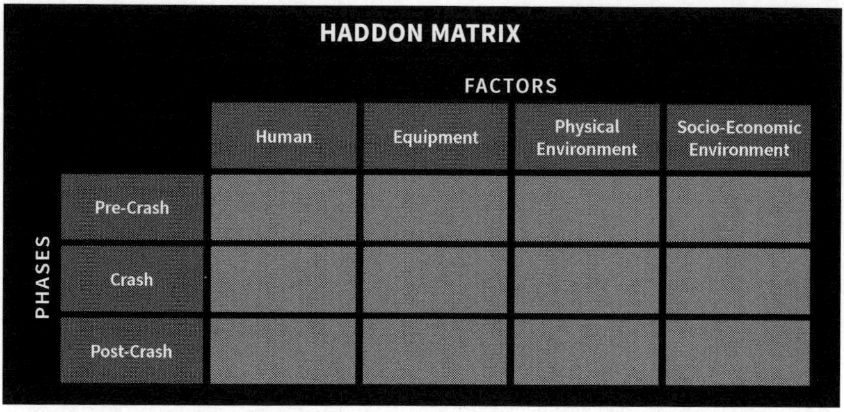

PHASES	FACTORS			
	Human	Equipment	Physical Environment	Socio-Economic Environment
Pre-Crash				
Crash				
Post-Crash				

HADDON MATRIX

Figure 3.2.[5] *The Haddon Matrix.*

Ralph Nader also appeared on the American scene in the mid-1960s. He gained prominence with his book *Unsafe at Any Speed*. With elaborate anecdotes and dramatic recreations of research by others and seasoned with depictions of legal actions, Nader brought consumer activists to the barricades. They seemed to view much of the road traffic tragedy to be the fault of Chrysler, Ford, General Motors and Volkswagen. Haddon had preceded Nader with more scholarly examinations of auto safety design deficiencies, but Nader raised the issue with the public.

Nader wielded influence. He was operating at the apex of government power on Capitol Hill. The Senate Commerce Committee took up the issue of regulating auto makers. Nader testified before the committee and national TV audiences in a media scramble. New regulations and standards were established. The National Traffic Safety Agency was formed in 1966, with Haddon as its first chief, to detail the regulations and to administer and enforce them.

Nader continued to be involved in the safety aspects of autos, later running for president of the United States four times. However, despite all of this action, road traffic deaths continued to increase in the United States and Western Europe.

The Highway Safety Act of 1966[6]

Since automobiles first appeared, America has never lacked overall safety and road traffic safety theorists and practitioners. The National Safety Council was formed in 1912 to aid in industrial safety, but quickly took on road and traffic related safety issues as traffic fatalities reached 30,000 annually and associated injuries increased proportionally. Until the establishment of the National Highway and Traffic Safety Administration (NHTSA), the council supplied key annual statistics in cooperation with the Federal Highway Administration (FHWA). Many state, regional and local traffic safety organizations emerged. These spawned varying degrees of safety experts, many of whom disregarded the classic test findings.

The very peak of authority and action concerning the entire road and highway infrastructure in the USA lies with the Committee on Transportation and Infrastructure of the US House of Representatives. Funding bills concerning roads and highways originate with this committee and are then passed to the companion Committee on the Environment and Public Works of the Senate. The chair of the House Committee and the ranking minority member, in addition to their regular offices, have private quarters in the committee suite in the Rayburn House Office Building across Independence Avenue from the Capitol. This building also includes staff offices and a large committee room for hearings and meetings. Almost every state with multiple representatives in Congress has a seat on this committee. It dispenses federal funds to the states to pay as much as 90% of the costs for construction and operation of the Interstate Highways and other roads of the United States Federal Aid Highway System. It also similarly aids railroads and expands or builds airports and seaports and is responsible for water resources. With the funding to the states, the committee imposes a significant degree of federal policy.

It was in this committee, then The Committee on Public Works, that the Highway Safety Act of 1966 took shape. The purpose of the act was to respond to the mounting increase in road traffic crashes and deaths. Under the leadership of Chairman George Fallon, Democrat of Maryland, the proposed law focused on remedies of improving driver behavior and performance. Provisions were included for: uniform standards of law and enforcement, mitigation of alcohol-impaired driving, driver education, licensing (including testing operating proficiency), physical and optical testing, keeping of crash records, crash investigations, vehicle registrations, road design and maintenance, traffic control, vehicle codes, emergency services, surveillance for high or potentially high crash locations and improving pedestrian performance. All but seven states were reported to have inadequate road safety programs, standards and action.

The bill further required every state to have a road safety program reflecting federal standards aimed at the sought-after performance improvements. Each state was required to have a Governor's Highway Safety Representative. The plan in the law was for these safety representatives to act as point persons in each state for coordinating the application of standards among the state police, highway, education and other responsible departments. They would also liaise with federal representatives of the Department of Transportation. Through these required standards, Congress and the Department of Transportation set a national safety program.

The staff of the committee, top professionals in their fields, with the Chairman and ranking members of both political parties, felt ownership in such legislation. The act was fully bipartisan. Action at the highest level was needed and it was taken. The act was delivered to the full House of Representatives for quick action and then sent to the Senate. After both passed the bill, President Lyndon Johnson signed it in September 1966.

It was a substantial plan that appeared to address all needed perceived deficiencies in traffic safety and to take all needed action to reduce fatalities and injuries. Some slowing of the growth in traffic crash tragedy seemed to emerge. Five years later, however, fatalities were still increasing and reached close to 53,000 in 1971, a level 45% higher than the number of fatalities recorded in 1961.[7] Unrestrained increases were still being forecast. Journalists called attention to different prospective causes. The results of the legislation were singularly disappointing.

A concept born in the Truman and Eisenhower annual conferences on road safety might explain the thinking of the time. The President's Committee on Traffic Safety reported 11 functions that the conferences considered necessary. These were:

- Laws and Ordinances
- Traffic Accident Records
- Education
- Engineering: Highway and Vehicles
- Motor Vehicle Administration: Driver Licensing and Motor Vehicle Inspection
- Police Traffic Supervision
- Traffic Courts
- Public Information
- Research
- Health, Medical Care and Transportation of the Injured
- Organized Citizen Support

In the philosophy behind the act was the idea that there was no panacea solution to reducing road traffic crashes. While this is true, priorities of action are critical. There was acceptance of what was labeled a "balanced approach" promoted in testimony by Howard Pyle, then President of the National Safety Council.[8] Others agreed. This led to scattered attempts rather than focusing on determining the right things to do first to produce results.

The National Traffic and Motor Vehicle Safety Act of 1966[9]

At about the same time as the House Public Works Committee began formulating the Highway Safety Act of 1966, the Senate Commerce Committee took up the National Traffic and Motor Vehicle Safety Act of 1966 under the leadership of chairman Warren

G. Magnuson. This was companion legislation "to provide for a coordinated national safety program and establishment of safety standards for motor vehicles in interstate commerce to reduce accidents involving motor vehicles and to reduce the death and injuries occurring in such accidents."[10] It was the first time the federal government in the United States seriously considered enacting national standards for vehicle safety. In his 1966 State of the Union address, then President Johnson called for action to "arrest the destruction of life and property on our highways."[11]

Federal standards had been proposed prior to this, but the big American automobile manufacturers had endeavored to prevent any such standards from becoming law. They instead favored self-regulation with voluntary industry standards. The act focused on providing basic safety standards that are now customary in the rich world. Effective for vehicles manufactured on or after January 1, 1968, the first standards included requirements for: front seat lap and shoulder seatbelts, collapsible steering columns, front seat head restraints, safer door latches and rear view mirrors. After the bill cleared the House with minor changes, the act was signed on the same day in September 1966 as the Highway Safety Act of 1966.

Neither of the 1966 acts, nor the philosophies of Haddon or Nader, suggested the need for priorities of action. However, the needs for such priorities were about to be realized in high-income nations. In 1972, American and Western European road traffic fatalities were still increasing.[12]

The Highway Safety Act of 1973[13]

Once again, the staff of the US House of Representatives Committee on Public Works, with the Federal Highway Administration road safety and traffic operations personnel, confronted the road safety issue and the seemingly unstoppable increases in traffic crashes and deaths. What else might be done to slow the growth in traffic tragedy and what had gone wrong with the actions from the Highway Safety Act of 1966? They faced the question of what was the main cause of crashes other than bad weather. Was it bad drivers, drunk driving or otherwise impaired drivers, unsafe cars or something else, like unsafe roads?

Looking for solutions, William (Bill) Harsha, Republican of Ohio and the Ranking Minority Member, with the assent of Chairman John Blatnik, Democrat of Minnesota, took the lead and gave orders for the staff to develop an omnibus highway safety bill. The staff was to look for countermeasures that might work and incorporate them in a bill for thorough review in committee hearings. The hearings would be open to all who had something to add to the discussion. It was hoped that new ideas would surface.

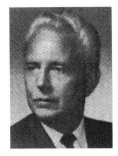

Figure 3.3.[14] *William H. Harsha 1973. Then Ranking Minority Member, Committee on Public Works, US House of Representatives.*

One such idea came from Potters Industries. The company, as related in Chapters 1 and 5, was conducting a series of tests of pavement marking in West Milford, New Jersey. Potters was then, and still is, the world leader in producing glass beads for reflectorizing pavement markings on roads.

Interested in expanding pavement marking in America, and knowing of its huge safety effectiveness indicated by the classic road marking tests discussed in Chapter 2, Potters executives contacted the House committee. They went through New Jersey Congressman Robert A. Roe, whose district included the township of West Milford. He referred them to Walter R. May, staff director for the Subcommittee on Investigation and Oversight, which was looking for technologies and ideas for the omnibus safety bill. May's curiosity was sparked. He asked that Potters provide him with everything that was known about pavement marking.

Potters created a dossier which featured the classic tests and the popular appeal of pavement markings. With this in hand, May referred Potters to Clifford Enfield, Minority Staff Director, and Richard C. Peet, Esq., Associate Minority Counsel. It was Dick Peet who did much of the preparation of the legislation for Bill Harsha. Committee Staff Director Richard Sullivan, and Assistant Lloyd Rivard, helped as needed at the behest of Chairman Blatnik. In those days, partisan relations in Congress were cordial, cooperative and productive.

The West Milford, NJ Tests

In the township of West Milford, one of the largest in New Jersey with 139 miles of roads, the Potters testing of pavement marking performance and durability also included demonstrations. The basic format was to paint one yellow center line with the standard composition: 15 mils thick (380 microns), 40 liters of paint per km (17 gallons per mile) and 0.7 kg of glass beads per liter (six pounds per gallon). Then a parallel line, as part of the dual center line, was a test or demonstration line. The lines were installed in

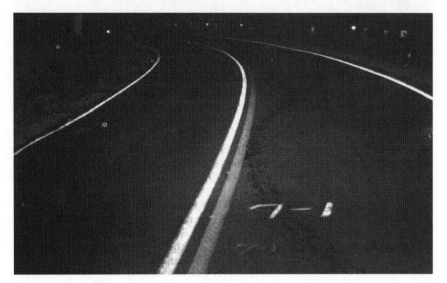

Figure 3.4.[15] *Parallel lines comparing a reflectorized center line (left) with an un-reflectorized center line (right) at night.*

test sections along the roads, all of which had respectable average daily traffic of 2,000 vehicles or more. The test sections were never less than 0.4 km (0.25 mile) long, with curves and hills. Parallel lines comparing a reflectorized line with an un-reflectorized line at night were one demonstration. Different thicknesses of paint, with different amounts of glass beads applied, were evaluated. So were different types of beads.

With this protocol, Potters established a new testing capability. The test was big, involving 32 kilometers (20 miles) of rural roads. From the beginning of pavement marking, testing of the durability and performance of longitudinal road markings, those parallel to

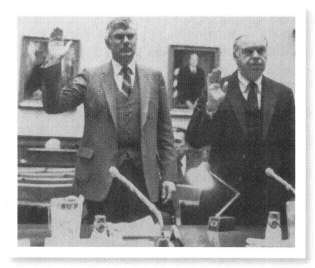

Figure 3.5.[16] *Gerry Balcar (co-author, left), Chief Marketing Officer and John Manley, President and Chief Operating Officer, both of Potters Industries, being sworn in to testify before the Subcommittee on Investigations and Oversight of the House Committee on Transportation and Infrastructure in 1981. This was follow-on testimony to the programs enacted by the Highway Safety Act of 1973.*

the traffic flow, was considered to be impossible because of the difficulty of recording changes in the test sections. Traditionally, tests of paint, thermoplastic, epoxy and other lines across the traffic flow was the only way to evaluate the length of time it took for markings to fail. The Potters solution was to run a movie camera over each test section every month. Eight designated evaluators were used to individually evaluate each section monthly and to record changes. In pavement marking research, this was a big step forward. Nobody had previously been able to document changes over time in longitudinal markings.

Potters executives and researchers invited Congressman Roe and the committee staff, the Senate Committee on Environment and Public Works staff and FHWA staff to visit the West Milford test site. There they also met visitors from Western European highway departments interested in the test. In road safety, this was a large and unique effort. Discussions about pavement marking and night driving issues ensued. Visitors got a full dose of the test by driving the test sections and experiencing the different markings firsthand.

Focusing on the safety aspects of the roads, the committee staff developed action programs of extending pavement marking, high hazard treatments, and roadside obstacle removal, as being means of achieving short-term crash reduction results. Such tested countermeasures had eluded them in preparing the Highway Safety Act of 1966. Now they saw that by making road safety improvements, quick results to stop the unnerving upward trend of roadway tragedy were possible.

Asked to give testimony in the committee hearings, Potters' researchers identified the key safety issue as being crashes on rural roads at night. An important initiative in 1967 by the Federal Highway Administration began the development of more detailed

	URBAN		RURAL	
	Fatalilties	Death Rate per 100 M Vehicle Miles Traveled	Fatalilties	Death Rate per 100 M Vehicle Miles Traveled
Day	8,200	1.9	17,400	4.3
Night	9,400	5.2	19,700	11.6
Total	17,600	2.9	37,100	6.5

FEDERAL HIGHWAY ADMINISTRATION'S DEATH RATE STATISTICS FOR 1971

Table 3.1.[17] *Data from the Federal Highway Administration presented by Potters Industries to the Subcommittee on Transportation of the Committee on Public Works, House of Representatives, Ninety-third Congress, First Session on H.R. 2332 to Authorize Appropriations for Certain Highway Safety Projects, and for other Purposes. March 6, 1973.*

data with fatalities tabulated by road system. Using data encompassing traffic counts, vehicle registrations, fuel consumption, and vehicle miles traveled, algorithms were tested and used to estimate the rates of fatalities per hundred million vehicle miles on each road system. Light condition was also a variable. It was found that two-thirds of the deaths were on rural roads, half of those at night. It became evident that it was six times more dangerous to drive on a rural two-lane road at night than on an urban two-lane road during the day. It seemed indeed that something might be wrong with the roads. Why would essentially the same drivers have six times more crashes with fatalities on rural roads at night? Films

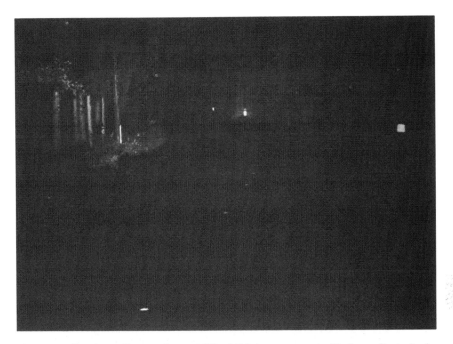

Figure 3.6.[18] *Union Valley Road, West Milford, NJ shown unmarked before reflectorized lines were installed.*

showing driving on unmarked rural roads at night compared to those with reflectorized center lines and edge lines were also convincing that road marking made a big difference. The concept of improving traffic safety by implementing road safety engineering, and hence including the roads in the safety equation, took shape.

In projecting possible reductions in crashes, injuries and fatalities, Potters leaned on the classic tests of markings, as did the committee staff. Potters also, with insight as to how much pavement marking was being done in the US, was able to show that 1.3 million km (800,000 miles) of America's paved federal-aid rural arterial and collector roads were unmarked or lacked edge lines. By marking these roads with center lines and edge lines, the projected decrease in road traffic fatalities was 8,000 annually.

The full Public Works committee voted out an initial draft of the new highway safety bill, HR 2332. Sponsored by Bill Harsha, and bearing the names of all 39 members of the committee as co-sponsors, Republicans and Democrats, it became the fully bipartisan

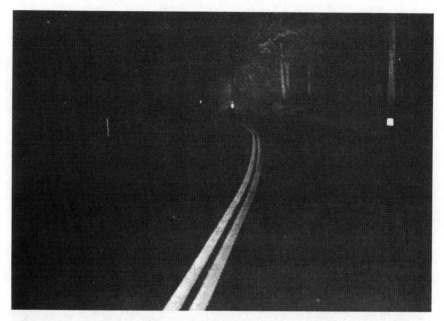

Figure 3.7.[19] *Union Valley Road, West Milford, NJ shown after the installation of reflectorized center lines.*

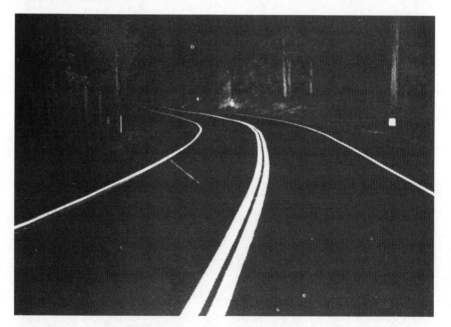

Figure 3.8.[20] *Union Valley Road, West Milford, NJ shown after the installation of reflectorized center lines and edge lines.*

Highway Safety Act of 1973. With this act, the staff created the Pavement Marking Demonstration Program, funded at $75 million per year. This was not nearly enough to install center lines and edge lines on all of the roads that were not marked. It was enough for the states, however, to test an adequate length of their unmarked roads to see for themselves what might happen. Thirty-eight states initially participated with all states eventually using the funds. Most reported very positive results that led to continued installation and maintenance of center lines and edge lines on their roads.

The test roads in West Milford, NJ had something more to contribute. During the period when America was deeply concerned over increasing road crashes, injuries and fatalities, the findings of the classic tests of edge lines were overlooked or ignored. Of course, the public hardly knew of these tests. Doubtful highway authorities and construction contractor lobbyists could refer to the one test (in Kansas, see Chapter 2) that failed to show any clear improvement in safety results.

Potters then sought to find an unmarked road in West Milford with an adequate average daily traffic count (ADT) that could be fully marked and tested with adjacent control roads left unmarked. One main road, 7.4 km (4.6 miles) long, had only an un-reflectorized white center line with no indicated passing zones. It also had 2.4 crashes per kilometer per year (3.9 per mile), with at least one fatality every year. County roads in the township had white reflectorized edge lines and a single white reflectorized center line without passing zones indicated. Other township roads had only un-reflectorized center line markings.

For the test, full reflectorized markings, white edge lines and all-yellow center lines with passing zones replaced the single un-reflectorized center line on the test road. The all-yellow reflectorized center lines with passing zones were painted on the test road on either side of the single white center line. All of the remaining collector roads of the town, 56 kilometers (35 miles) were the control roads. The test would extend for four months, May through August, in the summer with no winter conditions. With separate but nearby control roads, this test was similar in design to the classic test in Illinois.

- On the road that received full marking treatment for the first time, crashes decreased 44% compared to the average of the same months of the previous two years.
- Where passing zones were added, crashes decreased 15% versus the average of the same months of the previous two years.
- On the control roads, crashes increased 17% versus the average of the same months of the previous two years.

With this West Milford crash reduction test, the United States had a new test that updated and confirmed the German tests in Lower Saxony and Hesse with the added benefit of separate control roads. The results were as dramatic as the German tests of unmarked roads that had never been delineated. The results also supported the findings of all of the classic tests in America with the exception of the one Kansas test.[21]

Highlights from the Highway Safety Act of 1973

An analysis of where traffic deaths were occurring revealed that more than two-thirds were on rural roads. The act proposed four action programs focused on these rural roads. Three of these embodied a new concept of road safety engineering to improve the safety performance of roads. These were (1) the pavement marking demonstration program, (2) high hazard spot improvements and (3) obstacle removal. To prevent crashes, this safety engineering was to provide aid to drivers to help them avoid crashes and to eliminate road and highway hazards. The fourth action program was railroad crossing improvements by separating rail and road traffic with overpasses or underpasses and by adding warning lights or gates at grade crossings. The pavement marking demonstration program, however, was the centerpiece of the act.

Results from the West Milford tests proved that the safety effectiveness of pavement markings far outstripped the other action programs in reducing road crashes and deaths. Rail crossing separation and upgrading of warning devices would affect only the rail crossing sites. Similarly, high hazard treatment and obstacle removal were site specific. Center lines and edge lines work their safety effectiveness all along all the roads and highways.

The road-building contractors in the USA were shaken by the proposed use of Highway Trust Fund money for road safety purposes. Their view, which became a chorus from the state capitals,

THE SAFETY IMPROVEMENT PROGRAMS

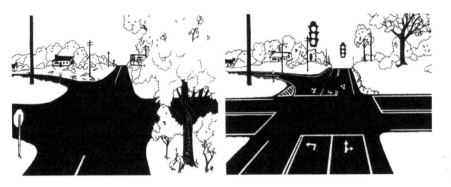

HIGH HAZARD IMPROVEMENTS AND OBSTACLE REMOVAL

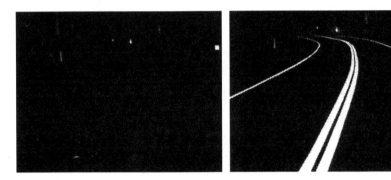

PAVEMENT MARKING

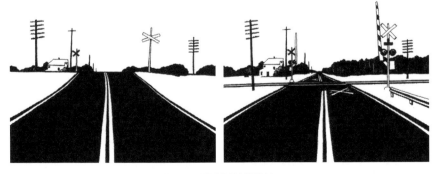

RAIL-HIGHWAY CROSSINGS

Figure 3.9.[22] *The Highway Safety Act of 1973 Road Safety Improvement Programs.*

was that increased road safety would be achieved only by rebuilding deficient roads or shifting traffic from surface streets to limited access interstate highways. Their dogma was that the money from the federal gasoline tax was to be used only for expansion of, and improvements to, the transportation infrastructure by building, maintaining or repairing roads or other structures. They voiced their objections. Bill Harsha told them the Highway Trust Fund money would be used for road safety engineering. Their very powerful lobbyists in Washington and in state capitols took action. They elucidated a protest on their behalf from the White House.

The high hazard treatment and obstacle removal actions that were supposed to be quick fixes, like adding signs and signals or clearing sight distances, emerged as construction projects to widen roads, add shoulders, straighten curves and level or re-grade hills. A fifth action program of bridge reconstruction or replacement "for reasons of improving safety" was added to provide road safety money for road construction contractors. But as the years passed, funds for the spot improvement and obstacle removal programs were allowed to be used for pavement marking. States could choose between road safety engineering and construction projects.

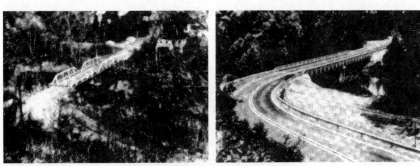

BRIDGE RECONSTRUCTION/REPLACEMENT

Figure 3.10.[23] *The Highway Safety Act of 1973 Bridge Reconstruction/Replacement Program.*

The classic tests and the West Milford tests foretold the results of the succeeding ten years after 1975. The members and staff of the then House Committee on Public Works, the Federal Highway Administration staff, and all others involved took comfort in the outcome.

The Road Safety Results

For comparison, 1973 is the baseline year before the implementation of the 1973 act. Events in 1973 were clearly not affected by the act. The center lines with passing zones, and edge lines, installed in annual increments, were largely completed by 1985 with a real national impact.

There was also the anomaly of the oil embargo in 1974. The response of Arab oil producing nations to the victory by Israel in the Yom Kippur War that began in October of 1973 was that oil exports to the United States and other allies of Israel were embargoed. Prices of gasoline shot upward and the reduced supplies brought memorable waiting lines at gas stations. Travel in the US was reduced in 1974 by 1.5%, only to increase again in 1975 and the years thereafter.[24] Road crashes and deaths were similarly reduced in 1974, only to edge up again after 1975.

The issue is, however, what were the results in the years from 1973 to 1985? There was a clear effect, led by the extensive increase of pavement markings on rural roads:

- On rural federal-aid roads, excluding the Interstate System, fatalities declined 35%.[25]
- On the urban portion of the federal aid roads, excluding the Interstate System, fatalities increased 17%.[26]
- In vehicle miles traveled, the federal-aid system carried 85% of the national total. During the period 1973-1985, vehicle miles traveled on rural roads, excluding Interstate roads, increased 17%. On urban streets and highways the increase was 87%.[27]

As a gasoline conservation measure, Congress enacted a 55 mile per hour (90 km per hour) national speed limit in 1974. Few rural roads, if any, on which the deaths were occurring, and that were to be newly marked with reflectorized lines, previously had a higher speed limit. Some on Capitol Hill heralded the action of the lower speed limit as a huge life saver. The reality was that it had little effect. Deaths on the Interstate System declined by 31% in 1974 compared to 1972. The net decrease was 1,514 fewer

FATALITIES
FEDERAL AID SYSTEM EXCLUDING INTERSTATE

YEAR	RURAL	URBAN	TOTAL	% RURAL
1973	25,227	11,398	36,625	68.88%
1974	20,373	10,053	30,426	66.96%
1975	20,178	10,490	30,668	65.79%
1976	18,788	11,078	29,866	62.91%
1977	19,721	11,214	30,935	63.75%
1978	20,602	12,200	32,802	62.81%
1979	20,487	13,286	33,773	60.66%
1980	19,689	13,898	33,587	58.62%
1981	19,061	13,890	32,951	57.85%
1982	16,918	12,497	29,415	57.51%
1983	15,964	12,415	28,379	56.25%
1984	16,539	13,172	29,711	55.67%
1985	16,305	13,311	29,616	55.05%
Change 1973-1985	-8,922	1,913	-7,009	
% Change 1973-1985	-35.4%	16.8%	-19.1%	

Source: FHWA

Table 3.2.[28] *Road Traffic Fatalities on the Federal Aid System, Excluding Interstate, 1973-1985.*

deaths.[29] How many deaths were due to reduced travel or reduced speed is uncertain.

Seatbelt use was in the early stages of driver acceptance and under 14% of drivers through 1984 used them, reaching 20% only in 1985.[30] Any contribution to saved lives as a result of seatbelt use during the 1973-1985 period is not clear. The strong efforts of Mothers Against Drunk Driving (MADD), igniting new interest in preventing driving while intoxicated, started only in 1980 with the group's founding by Candace Lightner. In 1982, the Presidential Commission on Drunk Driving lent forceful support to MADD's campaign. Statistics indicate that by 1985 there were already 3,000 fewer alcohol-related deaths on US roads compared to 1982.[31] Improved comprehensive emergency medical services ordained by the Highway Safety Act of 1966 were largely in place by 1975. Ongoing further improvements continued.

The Highway Safety Act of 1973 took note of new analyses of the road systems on which deaths and crashes occurred. This is relevant when the safety improvements on various road systems are the issue. The rural federal-aid secondary system and a portion of the primary system in America in 1972 were not given the most important safety treatment, namely center lines and edge lines. When this was completed in 1985 with the Pavement Marking Demonstration Program, the death rate per 100,000 population in the United States was brought down from 26.1 in 1972 to 18.4 in 1985.[32]

Subsequent to this, results from other targeted efforts aimed at single goals accrued as the population death rate was further reduced:

- Growing seatbelt use, reported to be 87% by 2013, brought increased survivability.[33] It was the result of a long campaign by activists and state governments passing laws requiring seatbelt buckling.
- The combined actions of Mothers Against Drunk Driving and The Presidential Commission on Drunk Driving, plus continued media coverage, legal enforcement and social pressure, resulted in less driving after drinking, and more designated drivers. Deaths resulting from alcohol impaired drivers were reduced from 21,000 in 1982 to 10,000 in 2013.[34]
- Crashworthiness of cars has continually improved with the use of crumple zones and other advancements.
- Emergency medical services, which serve more than just the needs of traffic crash victims, became fully available in most of the United States.

In 1971, the US House Committee on Public Works, led by Bill Harsha, John Blatnik, senior members and their notable staff, plus the staff of the Federal Highway Administration led by Director Lester Lamm, opened a new range of thinking about road traffic crash reduction. They established priorities of action and brought the effect of the safety condition of roads into the traffic safety equation. It was a huge step forward. The principle was to start with the known effectiveness of road safety engineering, and most importantly with reflectorized center lines and edge lines, to treat safety deficiencies of existing roads. This approach worked, even though at the time, no one involved realized fully what a momentous change they were bringing about.

In subsequent years, this was followed by targeted programs of promoting seatbelt use and of reducing impaired driving, which also worked. The new range of thinking led to getting roads up to the best possible safety standard as quickly as possible as a high priority. In the advanced concepts included in Vision Zero, getting the road system perfected is paramount.

The nations of Western Europe also found themselves struggling with rapidly increasing deaths and injuries on their roads in the 1960s. While recovering from World War II, most followed America's lead in implementing traffic crash reduction countermeasures. By 2013, the average population death rate of Western European countries was about five, less than half the US rate of 10.6.[35] What the Western European nations did differently to accomplish these results is discussed in our next chapter.

A Biographical Note for the American Story

The group that formed in 1971, at the behest of the US House of Representatives Committee on Public Works, did not realize at the time they were making road safety history with the profound changes in road safety thinking they proposed. Yet that is what they did by promulgating the Highway Safety Act of 1973. The initiative came from William Harsha, Ranking Minority Member, looking for means to curb the increases in road traffic fatalities ongoing for a decade. With the assent of Committee Chairman John Blatnik, the staff of the Subcommittee on Investigations and Oversight was activated to look for new road traffic crash countermeasures or other new ideas. Walter May was the staff director of the subcommittee. George Kopecky was Deputy and Technical Advisor. The subcommittee Chairman was James Wright, who later became Speaker of the House. Chief Counsel, Richard Sullivan and his technical advisor Lloyd Rivard, joined in the search for promising ideas. Richard C. Peet, Esq., Associate Minority Counsel, did the overall job of putting the law together, coordinating the hearings, drafting reports, and general oversight working with Minority Staff Director Cliff Enfield. Dorothy Beam and Erla Yeomans were the Executive Staff Assistants giving administrative and other support.

On the senate side, Peter Domenici was Chairman of the Subcommittee on Transportation of the Committee on Environment and Public Works. Clark Norton was his staff director. From the Federal Highway Administration, Robert Connor, Clark Bennett, and Howard Anderson, all senior professionals, influenced developments with Lester Lamm, the Director.

As events progressed in 1975, and beyond with reauthorization of the act, congressmen James Howard and E. G. "Bud" Shuster, who both became committee chairmen, assumed roles as did Salvatore D'Amico and Clyde Woodle who later became staff directors. They were supporters who kept road safety action moving along.

New Jersey congressman Robert A. Roe played a key role introducing Potters Industries to the committee of which he also became chairman. Glenn Johnson was his administrative assistant and staff chief. Potters Industries became a main source of road safety data and Roe lent continued support to the company's extensive road testing and historical research efforts. Involved from Potters Industries, aside from co-author Gerry Balcar, CMO, were Thomas K. Wood, Chairman and CEO; John Manley, President and COO; Timothy O'Leary, Vice President Sales; James Ritter, Technical Director and Anita Ward, Marketing Research Manager.

The committee staff also asked for the help of the 3M Company, then the Minnesota Mining and Manufacturing Company, principal producers of, and leading experts in, reflective road signing of all types worldwide and of other road safety products. Andrew Lampe was the executive representative.

The township of West Milford, New Jersey provided its roads to the Potters Industries' tests. The local government became involved. The mayor was Charles DeLade who greeted many guests from Washington, other states and from Europe and Japan. Robert Little, Edward Gola and John Andresan were on the town council and joined Mayor DeLade in greeting visitors. Peter Roan was the

Town Manager. James Breslin was police chief; James Dykstra and John Way were senior officers. Anthony Buzzoni was the township engineer. Adrian Birdsall was in charge of road marking. Host to visitors was Carl Masen at his memorable hotel and restaurant.

In the aggregate effort, which indeed changed road safety thinking, Bill Harsha was the leader who developed a deep personal knowledge of road safety and the new theory which became road safety engineering. Dick Peet marshaled the theory into the necessary details and was the chief coordinator and communicator. He and Harsha made things happen. Bob Connor was the essential contact with the Federal Highway Administration with the latest research information, ideas and support. He was the de-facto chief traffic engineer of the United States. Both Bob Conner and Dick Peet were visitors to West Milford several times as were Congressman Roe and Glenn Johnson. Almost everyone else involved visited West Milford at least once.

4

The Western European Story

The principal nations of Western Europe in 1945 faced the re-establishment of their governments and financial systems after World War II. German cities had been bombed into rubble, other areas were ruined by intense warfare. The national economies of the combatants were in shambles. Hard fighting had swept across Belgium, France, Italy and the Netherlands, causing widespread destruction. Those nations plus Austria, Denmark, Luxembourg, and Norway had suffered Nazi occupation. Britain was victorious but bankrupt. Only Ireland, Portugal, Spain, Sweden and Switzerland were unscathed, with only commercial losses.

After World War II, the Allies did not make the mistakes of 1918-1919. The comprehensive Bretton-Woods Agreement of 1944 at the 44 nation *United Nations Monetary and Financial Conference,* established new, stable and enforceable currency exchange rates. These prevented competitive revaluations by the European states and overvalued the US dollar to attract investment into Europe from America. The Agreement also founded the *International Bank for Reconstruction and Development* (IBRD), which later became *The World Bank*, to make long-term capital available to nations urgently needing foreign aid. The *International Monetary Fund* (IMF) was also established to manage exchange rates and keep them within bounds. All of this proved helpful, but was not enough. The United States added The Marshall Plan in 1947, which provided more billions of dollars across Europe. Economic growth ignited, sometimes exceeding 10% per year in some nations. Some economies doubled in size in less than a decade.

The life of the auto age, which originated in Europe, soon resumed in earnest. The beginning of growing roadway tragedy became evident in startling statistics. As in America, increases were such that by 1972, the road traffic death rates per 100,000 population were comparably as high as those in some low- and middle-income countries in 2013. In Germany, the rate was 27.0; in France it was 35.2; in Italy, 22.1; in the Netherlands, 24.6; in Austria, 40.2; in Denmark, 22.4. The rates were lower in a victor nation, the United Kingdom, where it was 14.5. In noncombatant Sweden and Spain, it was 14.7 and 16.9 respectively. In Ireland it was 21.2. The United States registered 26.1, but had the money and expertise, it was assumed, to effectively deal with the problem.[1]

Adopting Road Safety Engineering

With increasing fatalities on their roads, the highway authorities of Western Europe, and its recovering professional or activist road safety establishment, looked to the United States for leadership. The increases in road traffic fatalities beginning in the 1960s could not be restrained. For two decades, developments to combat increasing road traffic crashes and deaths were parallel in the United States and Western Europe, focusing on efforts to change driver and pedestrian behavior.

By popular demand, center lines were reinstalled on Western European roads as before the war. Western European drivers, like their American counterparts, were delighted with the reflectorized lines. When edge lines appeared, they were as popular as in America. After the passing of the American Highway Safety Act of 1973, the whole road traffic safety issue shifted quickly to include roads and their safety potential in a new approach from Capitol Hill in Washington. The same attitude was soon adopted in the capitals of Western Europe. Use of road safety engineering, and particularly for reflectorized center lines and edge lines, emerged. A measure of this success was traceable to the events in Washington described in Chapter 3.

Specialists in transport at Western European embassies in the American capital had followed the development of the Highway Safety Act of 1966, the huge program that tried to stem increases in road traffic crashes, injuries and deaths. Then in 1973, as road safety engineering featuring the pavement marking idea made its way toward being passed by the US Congress, it also edged into diplomatic channels. With it came the new concept that roads were part of the traffic safety equation. The thinking that roads could be made safer, and crashes reduced, by installing reflectorized center lines and edge lines, and by improving intersections and rail crossings, became the ruling philosophy in most Western European highway departments.

Just as some in Washington objected to inaugurating road safety engineering, there were likewise naysayers in Western Europe. The latter claimed that refashioning behavior was the necessary and only way to reduce road traffic crashes and fatalities. If money was to be spent on road safety, those pursuing the traditional thinking of improving road user behavior wanted it for their road safety programs. It was soon clear, however, that those who overlooked the results of the classic road crash reduction tests described in Chapter 2 were wrong. The authorities in Western European nations responsible for the safety of the roads mostly followed the American lead.

Pavement marking was initially viewed in Western Europe as an American technology. American equipment was imported into Western Europe in the 1950s when the drivers started to ask for reflectorized markings like those in America. Center lines and edge lines were installed in and near cities. Every nation purchased striping trucks, or their pavement marking contractors did, to supply pavement marking services. American firms established branches in Western Europe. The earliest of the classic tests of road traffic crash and death reduction by adding pavement markings to rural roads were performed in Germany as noted in Chapter 2.

Within the road operations community in America, most attention was paid to the new Interstate Highways, urban streets and main rural arteries. Minor arteries and collector roads in rural areas were not usually marked with reflectorized center lines and edge lines prior to 1973, as was also true in Western Europe. The first discovery of the unusually high fatality rate per hundred million vehicle miles traveled on rural roads was determined in the United States (see Chapter 3). That started people realizing the effect of road conditions on crashes. Authorities in Western Europe grasped the idea of marking rural roads, recognizing there were more road traffic crashes and deaths on them.

As highway budgets were drawn, there proved to be a distinct geographic advantage in Western Europe. The distances between cities and for commutes to offices, factories or rail stations were a fraction of those in the United States. Less paint or thermoplastic, glass beads, motor fuel and labor time were needed. The costs to fully provide road traffic crash reductions in Western Europe were much lower than in the United States. The installation of center lines and edge lines on most of the roads in Western Europe was also completed much faster than in the USA. In the northern European nations with severe winters, thermoplastic came into early use in order to assure that lines would still be functional in the spring.

Western European Advances in Pavement Marking

As broad interest in pavement marking took hold in Western European highway departments, crash reduction results in the United States supported those who wanted to mark all significant roads with center lines and edge lines. Many nations began organizing striping trucks and work forces. As the need for ongoing maintenance of the lines expanded, pavement marking contractors took on more of this work. The emerging use of private contractors to do the marking brought the need for detailed, formal specifications when lines are newly installed and to set limits on wear. Moreover, it was recognized that the lines had to have a required minimum level of retroreflectivity to be effective.

Testing with wider lines, particularly edge lines, was a Western European initiative. The typical 10 cm wide line (4 inch) in America came to Western Europe with American equipment. It was not long before Western European engineers, highway department managers and others were wondering if the visual signal given by the narrow lines to drivers was a bit anemic. They began installing 15 cm (6 inch) and 20 cm (8 inch) lines, with a supportive response by the public. More detailed testing was to come in the United States with the results published by the Federal Highway Administration (see Chapter 5).

The many actions regarding standards and specifications for retroreflective markings created another issue. Was the yellow center line established in America to indicate opposite direction traffic on the other side of the line so important as to justify the lower visibility of retroreflectivity? After all, is it not obvious in a system of all white lines which ones are the center lines? "Not to everyone," said the Americans. The one driver in a thousand not understanding it can easily cause a crash. And, the Americans continued, a randomized survey of drivers who had driven in an all-white system and who were offered yellow lines on some of their roads, chose the latter overwhelmingly.

There is no clear answer to this issue. A very large research program, known as COST 331, was subsequently undertaken under the auspices of the European Commission to find optimal visibility standards for pavement marking in the European Union.[2] It also validated the use of lines wider than 10 cm (4 inch). It did not, however, set uniformity of road marking design throughout the European Union.

Highway authorities in Western Europe also had to deal with the skeptics who wondered if road safety engineering really made a difference. Some skeptics were fiscally motivated and retorted that too much of the information about crash reduction came from the private sector in the United States. The crash and death reduction results that materialized as rural roads were marked in America, however, were convincing. There was a clear reduction in crashes and fatalities when these roads were marked with center lines and edge lines. The results were further verified by the states conducting additional crash and fatality reduction tests on newly marked roads. Some other skeptics were the deniers. Reducing crashes, injuries and deaths with road safety engineering really was not dealing with the problem of poor driver and pedestrian behavior. Was there a lasting road safety effect with road safety engineering? It was for the future theorists of the "safe system" approach and Vision Zero to understand the long-term relationships.

Within a few years after 1973, Western Europe was for the most part fully center lined and edge lined, meaning that nearly all arterial and collector roads were marked and the lines regularly maintained. Conscious that road conditions affect overall road safety, the highway authorities of Western Europe took action with easy-to-do safety engineering improvements. Actions by the traditional road safety community were also successful. Alcohol-impaired driving is now minimal in most Western European nations and seatbelts are mostly buckled. All require the use of motorcycle, moped and bicycle helmets. There are also comprehensive driver licensing standards, universal driver training, vehicle safety specifications and inspections, separate lanes for bicycles and safety education and promotion.

Successes in Discouraging Drinking and Driving

With evident progress toward mitigating the serious levels of traffic crashes, injuries and deaths, the issues of seatbelt use and alcohol impaired driving were next to be confronted. In every country, the campaigns began to encourage, or require, buckling of seatbelts and discourage any drinking before driving.

In France, the counter drinking and driving campaign built up to a large national program supported strongly by the Elysee Palace. An inter-ministerial council was started, chaired by the prime minister. Then President Nicolas Sarkozy added new provisions upgrading the legal structure, including the introduction of alcoholism rehabilitation programs. As more of the drivers charged with Driving Under the Influence (DUI) offenses were those afflicted with alcoholism, a greater focus on treatment of that condition evolved.

Random breath tests are allowed in France with close to nine million reported in 2007.[3] As proof of the changing social norms regarding drinking and driving, a survey of about 4,800 young drivers (18-25 years of age) in eight European Union countries showed that 92% of young French drivers considered asking one person in a party to abstain from drinking to be the designated driver.[4] A reason for this high number might be that confiscation of a car can be a penalty if someone is caught impaired while driving. Compared to other Western European countries, France was slow in addressing drinking and driving but is more recently doing more. In 2012 for example, France enacted a law requiring a working breathalyzer in every car on the road for self-testing.[5]

In every Western European country, campaigns to discourage drinking before driving began. These were supported by laws tighter than in the USA and with more severe penalties. The allowable blood alcohol content (BAC) limits were often lower by half. Where in the United States, the BAC was at 0.1% at the time, in the two countries with the lowest fatality rates (Sweden and the United Kingdom), they were 0.05% and 0.08% BAC respectively.[6] These efforts, coupled with rigorous enforcement, brought universal results that were quickly adopted throughout Western Europe.

The United Kingdom established an ongoing anti drinking and driving television campaign in the mid-1960s. There was much publicity indicating how little some people, like 110-pound women, could drink before registering higher than the legal BAC limit. The general theme that four single whiskeys, about 1.6 dl (5.5 fl oz), would double the chances of a traffic crash continued in the campaign over two generations. Featured in the BBC 50th anniversary television ad of the campaign was the fact that going to prison for a crash caused by alcohol-impaired driving would seriously interfere with employment opportunities. This was the centerpiece of the UK effort for 50 years and is still being innovated and updated.

Early on, people went by taxi or hired car to dinner parties in London or Edinburgh. In the country, if taxis or for-hire cars were not available, dinner parties became house parties and guests stayed overnight. It became socially unacceptable to take a chance on causing a crash and injuries by driving under the influence. It was a social stigma to receive a summons for DUI, and much worse to be involved in a mishap. Likewise, just driving after drinking was socially an issue. It was simply not to be done, and using designated drivers became the norm. A host, hostess or friend asked for the car keys of someone who should not drive and sometimes arranged for overnight accommodations. Enforcement was part of the solution. In 1972, there were over 57,000 convictions of DUI in the United Kingdom, four times as many as in 1966.[7]

By the early 1970s, the same conditions existed in Sweden. A conviction or summons for DUI was a social stigma which few chose to risk. It also became acceptable for a host or hostess to ask for car keys and to arrange a bed. Families and guests took taxis to a restaurant and for the return trip. Enforcement was also strict. A first offense with a BAC of 0.1%, which was the former legal limit in the United States, could result in two years in jail. Being over the current low rate of 0.02% could mean six months in prison. Random breath testing was authorized, about 6,800 such tests per day, or 2.5 million per year, being reported in 2011.[8] These procedures resulted in a veritable net in which impaired drivers were caught. Repeat offenses could mean not only losing the privilege to drive, but also losing the car.

Random breath tests are not authorized in Germany. The minimum fine for a first DUI offense, however, is €500 (US $540) with a one month license suspension. A high BAC level over the 0.05% limit may result in a two year license suspension. If a crash involves personal injury or death, anyone arrested can expect to be fined and serve jail time in addition to license suspension or revocation and to have his or her car confiscated.[9] Fines and legal expenses can exceed €15,000 (US $16,000) as extensive and lengthy recertification tests are required to regain driving privileges.[10] Severe enforcement in Britain, Sweden and other countries supports social pressures and prospective social stigmas. In Germany, the pressure may be social, but it is also very much fear of the consequences in dealing with the police and the courts.

An unexpected, but successful, television campaign by the Belgian government called "Bob" developed, appearing in 1995 and aimed at getting people to use designated drivers. A series of television sketches about drinking and driving with doable solutions, it moved quickly into Luxembourg, France, the Netherlands and Germany. Large percentages of young people in Belgium responded to a survey in 2014 showing that 34% of the respondents had been designated drivers and 46% had been driven home by designated drivers.[11]

Seatbelt Use Laws and Campaigns

Beginning with Sweden, Spain and Finland in 1975, every major Western European country, except Italy, established seatbelt use laws before the first state in America did (New York in 1984). Laws also required seatbelts to be made available in cars, the United States being the first country to require these in 1965. This was followed in 1974 by a requirement for cars having three-point seatbelts. The major Western European nations followed suit. All new vehicles in Western Europe had three-point seatbelts soon thereafter.[12] The problem was how to get drivers and passengers to use them.

The campaigns and legislation for seatbelt use ran parallel to the anti drinking and driving efforts, which both started while road safety engineering programs were being completed, both meeting with similar success. Western European governments had a significant advantage over America in that they owned major broadcasting networks. In Britain, BBC was dominant. In France there were for a while only two government television channels. Germany also had government-owned regional broadcast outlets. Every nation had at least one government-owned network.

In Britain, the BBC carried television spots with realistic crash situations that often showed a passenger with a buckled seatbelt walking away from a crash while one not restrained gets taken away bleeding in an ambulance or is shown dead at the scene. Another clever characterization of unrestrained impact in a moving vehicle likened hitting the windshield in a crash to jumping off a building. An award-winning television spot showed a wife and daughter grabbing hold of the husband/father in a pantomime of an auto crash when he was not wearing a seatbelt. Another showed an unbelted rear seat passenger injuring a belted driver with a head impact. All pointed out that not wearing a seatbelt broke the law.

In Germany, enforcement of the buckle-up law was joined to television promotions with violent crashes pictured. In some, death is depicted by a spirit leaving an unbelted body or staying in a safely restrained one. Staged crashes showed the physics of being unrestrained with dummies' heads going through windshields. Much attention was given to how the unbelted are smashed around the interior of a car in a high-speed crash, injuring those who are wearing their seatbelts. An Italian ad shows numerous crashes in a one-minute spot speaking of the fatal consequences, or of disabling injury, in a simple crash when not using seatbelts. There was also one with a belted driver surviving seven rollovers when forced off a highway by a multi-vehicle collision.

Compared to other rich countries, the United States still has a lot of work to do in persuading its citizens to wear seatbelts while driving.

SEATBELT USE % SELECT COUNTRIES 2011		
COUNTRY	FRONT SEAT	REAR SEAT
Australia	97.0	92.0
Canada	95.5	89.2
Germany	98.0	97.0
Japan	97.0	63.7
Netherlands	96.6	82.0
Spain	87.7	79.5
Sweden	96.0	87.0
United Kingdom	96.0	90.5
United States	84.0	70.0

Source: WHO Global Health Observatory Data Repository

Table 4.1.[13] *Seatbelt use percentage for select countries 2011.*

Driver Licensing

A driver's license for the European Economic Area (EEA, the European Union plus Iceland, Lichtenstein and Norway), has replaced previous European licenses. It is a plastic card, sometimes with a chip, similar to a credit card, and is issued by each nation according to its requirements, renewable every ten years. The national requirements may vary but most stipulate that all applying for a first driver's license must attend a driving school and pass a two-stage test. The minimum age for a non-commercial vehicle license is 17, but it is 18 in most countries.

Driving schools are authorized by the licensing authorities of each nation, their instructors also being certified. There are national associations of the driving schools in each country as well. Training drivers is a specialized field in Western Europe, which has risen to the level of a post-secondary education discipline. The curriculum for new drivers includes 20 to 40 hours of instruction on traffic laws and 6 to 20 hours of practical driving instruction. Some nations require up to 3,000 kilometers (1,800 miles) of student driving before granting the license. All is overseen by a European-wide association that sets new standards and keeps instruction compatible with car designs. Regular academic educational authorities are not involved and educational time in traditional schools is not used. Nor is any money for driver training contained in typical education budgets. Driving schools are in the purview of traffic authorities alone.

Not only is it harder to become a new driver in Western Europe than in the United States, you also have to wait longer for the privilege. One observation is that if Western European practices were installed in America, there would be up to six million fewer drivers under the age of 18 in the USA. In 2009, of the fatal road traffic crashes in the United States, drivers aged under 25 were involved in 22% of them.[14] In the European Union, drivers aged 18 to 24 were in 17% of fatal road traffic crashes.[15]

The Lower Western European Fatality Rates

There remain questions of why the Western European population fatality rates now average less than half the American rate. There are some special facts and observations to explain this:

- The United States has significantly more vehicles per population than Western Europe.
- The United States is three times the size of Western Europe. There is significantly more rural travel on two-lane roads. Enforcement is more difficult over longer distances and so is road upkeep. American drivers spend more time on their roads, and travel twice as far every year, than their Western European counterparts.
- Western European governments, with their large and well-financed public broadcasting networks, have a communications advantage. Being the principal payer, they can broadcast safety messages freely and need not be concerned by any content they choose. They can push out messages and then evaluate the result.
- The allowable BAC level in the United States for driving

under the influence (0.08%) is higher than in most Western European nations, where the common level is 0.05%. Denmark and the Netherlands have low population death rates with a 0.05% BAC limit while Norway and Sweden using 0.02% are other low-population death rate countries. These countries and others also have strong social pressures against risking a DUI summons or worse.

- There are also fewer young drivers in Western Europe. While getting a learner's permit is a rite of passage to young Americans as young as age 14, it is not the same in Western Europe, where the license requirements are much more stringent. Attendance at expensive driving schools is mostly required. Insurance is also expensive. Moreover, rail transit or other modes of transport are generally available, inexpensive and convenient. At a minimum, new drivers in Western Europe are at least two years older than those in America.

- The critical variables may be law enforcement and social- and culture-related pressures. As well as the examples already given: In Italy, the first offense can go up to a fine of €2,000 (US $2,200) and a six-month license suspension with a BAC between 0.05% and 0.08%. More expensive and stringent penalties yet above 0.08% BAC. In Norway, where the BAC limit is 0.02%, an offense can carry a fine equal to one and a half month's base salary but not less than NOK 10,000 (US $1,250) if the BAC is over 0.05%. In the United Kingdom, the fine for a first offense can be £5,000 (US $7,800). In France, the fine can reach €4,500 (US $4,800), two years in prison and a three-year license suspension. Compared to most American states, these measures are very harsh. Researchers find them to be effective supplements to the social taboos. They have also found that impaired drivers remaining on the roads are mostly confirmed alcoholics.[16]

Then we can also compare the United States with Australia and Canada. These two large Commonwealth nations both have a BAC of 0.08% as the legal limit where impaired driving is presumed, the same as the USA. They also have lower population fatality rates than the United States, 5.7 and 6.0 respectively, the rate in the US being 10.7, for 2012.[17] Australia allows random breath testing. Fines for the first offense of driving over the limit are AUS $550 (US $405) to AUS $3,000 (US $2,220) and license suspension of at least six months.[18]

Canada also has tough enforcement. The first offense draws a fine of CAN $1,000 (US $770) and a one year driving prohibition. For a second offense, there is jail time and a two-year suspension of driving privilege.[19]

COMPARISON OF FATALITY RATES AND LEGAL BAC % LIMITS

COUNTRY	FATALITY RATE PER 100K POP. 1972	FATALITY RATE PER 100K POP. 2012	LEGAL BAC % LIMIT 2015	FATALITY RATE PER BILLION VEHICLE KM 1972	FATALITY RATE PER BILLION VEHICLE KM 2012
Austria	40.2	6.3	0.05	109.1	6.9
Belgium	32.0	6.9	0.05	94.9	7.7
Denmark	22.4	3.0	0.05	43.1	3.4
Finland	25.0	4.7	0.05		4.7
France	35.2	5.8	0.05		
Germany	27.0	4.4	0.05		5.0
Greece	12.9	8.9	0.05		
Iceland	11.1	2.8	0.05		2.9
Ireland	21.2	3.5	0.05	48.9	3.4
Italy	22.1	6.3	0.05		
Luxembourg	31.0	6.5	0.05		
Netherlands	24.6	3.4	0.05	54.4	4.4
Norway	12.5	2.9	0.02		3.3
Portugal	24.8	6.8	0.05		
Spain	16.9	4.1	0.05		
Sweden	14.7	3.0	0.02	29.3	3.7
Switzerland	26.8	4.3	0.05	52.4	5.6
United Kingdom	14.5	2.8	0.08		3.6
Australia	26.0	5.7	0.05		5.5
Japan	19.3	4.1	0.03	79.7	7.2
New Zealand	24.1	6.9	0.05		7.7
Canada	28.0	6.0	0.08		6.1
United States	26.1	10.7	0.08	27.1	7.0

Source: IRTAD and IARD

Table 4.2.[20] *Fatality rates and BAC % limits for 23 high-income OECD countries.*

Vision Zero

Out of the earlier and separate successes with road safety engineering, and the follow-on successes with reductions in drunk-driving, increased seatbelt use, driver regulation and educational and promotional programs, came the concept of Vision Zero in the late 1990s. The goal is to have no road fatalities or severe injuries as a human cost of having a modern automotive society. The idea originated in Sweden, the first country to reach a fatality rate per 100,000 population of under three. Now Denmark, Iceland, Ireland, the Netherlands, Norway, and the United Kingdom all have accomplished fatality rates below four.

The Vision Zero concept anticipates a perfected road system for all road users. Road safety engineering is an existing first step. The road is part of the grand solution for safer mobility and safety is considered a precondition for mobility. Where travel occurs is fundamental to the road safety equation. The road system should be made as safe as possible to accommodate for human mistakes as there will always be drivers who are fatigued, distracted, or otherwise impaired.

Vision Zero includes a safety culture concept that keynotes shared societal, industrial and individual responsibility. That means pedestrians, bicyclists and motorcyclists are careful and motorists avoid driving impaired and obey laws.

Another idea is that of livable cities. This concept aims to minimize the need for auto travel and instead promote public transport, walking, and bicycle use. This concept envisions easy access for getting to work, shopping and services.

The Western European story saw these nations attack increasing road traffic crashes and fatalities with the new philosophy of road safety engineering and carried that beyond its American dimensions. The principle of a "perfected road system" is a sound basis for advanced thinking. With road safety engineering in place and maintained, it provides an ongoing, basic reduction in road traffic crashes and deaths. Behavior countermeasures then add to these results. With Vision Zero and a "safe system" approach, Western Europe is leading the world in the next phase in advancing road safety.

5

Advances in Thinking about Road Marking

The classic road marking tests, and the success in America and Western Europe in the use of center lines and edge lines, were the beginning of the chronicle of pavement marking. Some of the new research and thinking that evolved was related to the science of vision from the driver's perspective. Other work concentrated on the use of wider lines, of measuring retroreflective signals and on the time needed by drivers to respond to what they see.

The Concept of Driver's Vision

The twentieth century leader of this vision related research was Professor Merrill Allen of the University of Indiana, noted for his innovative and probing work. He was fascinated by optics and vision as any leader in his discipline would be, but he added to that an equivalent fascination with driving, its visual requirements and its inherent obstacles to vision. On these subjects he became a recognized international authority.

Allen sought improvement in automotive windshield and hood designs and coatings. He found that tempered glass in some shapes could interfere with clear vision. He also found the glare of the sun, or bright lights at night, on car's hoods could impede the vision of drivers. He developed means to show what that kind of interference could do under various light conditions. Among his research tools were cars without windshields and/or with black felt hoods to absorb any glare. He tested the ability of drivers in a test course to see various potential or real immediate troubles using a "squeeze-when-seen" device similar to visual field tests which ophthalmologists use when evaluating glaucoma patients. Allen's test drivers rode the course in cars with various windshields, their performance being compared to what they saw in the car with no windshield. It was in those test cars that Allen would demonstrate how one really sees while driving.

In another experiment, Allen's team split about 5,000 cars into two approximately equal groups, a test group and a control group. On the front of the test cars, 25 candle-power lights were installed and turned on during daylight driving. On tabulation some months later, this group had 23% fewer crashes than the cars without the lights. As a result, it is a legal requirement in many countries to drive with daylight running lights, which are lights automatically turned on and then stay on all the time. Even in America, more people now drive with headlights on all the time.

Allen was adept at bringing in research grants or research cooperation. He was also a motivator looking for new ways to solve issues and brilliant in every way.

Allen's view was that vision was the source of 90% of the information needed to perform the task of driving. He wrote that good visual acuity, good peripheral vision, color sensitivity, night vision and glare recovery were needed. He indicated that much of the needed information comes from peripheral vision. Driving, he said, uses peripheral vision the way walking uses peripheral vision. Drivers drive with the edge of the road, or whatever is on the edge of the road like parked cars, as the key guide in the periphery. This alignment of the vehicle in the driving lane is guided continuously by the driver's peripheral vision. Edge lines and center lines are continuous signals to aid the driver's peripheral vision. For safe driving, Allen found edge lines and center lines essential.[1]

Foveal (center-eye) vision, in Allen's thinking, is used to target destinations, read signs and signals and to spot trouble. At highway speeds, if foveal vision time is used up positioning the vehicle on the road, there will not be enough vision time to deal with potential trouble that might pop up. That trouble could be difficulties seeing pedestrians or animals, for example, or dealing with another vehicle making an unexpected maneuver. Of all crashes that occur, Allen had data showing that 50% resulted from the driver not acquiring information fast enough.[2]

Allen saw night driving as particularly challenging, when typical peripheral guide devices are obscured. He saw reflectorized edge lines as vitally important. In daylight, the edge of the road is generally clear and continuous in peripheral vision. At night it can be hard to see and might take up foveal time. Drivers will use foveal vision in driving, as in walking, if they are uncomfortable about their ability to keep the car properly in the driving lane. Allen often made the point that only reflectorized center lines and edge lines will provide the needed continuous signal to peripheral vision from the periphery.

An illustration Allen used to test the reliance on peripheral vision while driving was with drivers at various levels of inebriation. He postulated that someone walking at a level of inebriation bumps into walls, doorways or furniture because peripheral vision is impaired. He said the same was true in driving except then the results could be an injury or a fatal crash. He cited these effects from alcohol impairment:[3]

- Lower contrast sensitivity makes spotting trouble more difficult
- Less flexible searching strategy (drivers look at fewer items on the roadway)
- "Tunnel vision" is evidenced when much in the periphery is lost
- Loss of dynamic visual acuity make images seen look blurred
- An early effect from alcohol impairment is narrowed peripheral vision
- Shortened visibility distances

If all of these vision issues were related to alcohol and driving, the questions had to come up: How many of the crashes and deaths prevented by edge lines and center lines, in the experience on America's rural roads and elsewhere, involved impaired drivers? Are not the impairment of peripheral vision or reduced contrast sensitivity countered by good center lines and edge lines? Are not tunnel vision or reduced distance vision likewise aided by center lines and edge lines? It seemed important to find out.

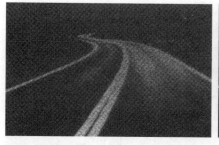

Contrast sensitivity is lowered. *To alcohol impaired drivers, shades of color tend to merge so that it is difficult to differentiate items in the road environment from one another.*

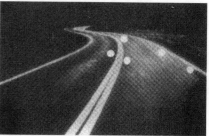

Search patterns are reduced. *Impaired drivers look at fewer items in the roadway, and hence obtain less information on which to base decisions.*

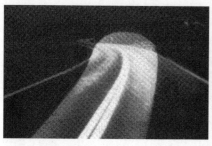

Peripheral vision is narrowed. *This compounds the difficulties of impaired drivers to maintain full visual contact with the road.*

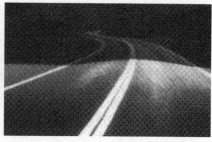

Visibility distance is shortened. *Impaired drivers tend to see only the roadway immediately in front of the vehicle. This allows less time for drivers to anticipate or react to potential problems or to make correct decisions.*

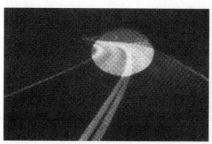

"Tunnel Vision" is evidenced. *Features of the roadside are not clear to impaired drivers.*

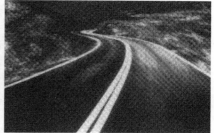

Dynamic visual acuity is lowered. *Separate items, particularly at the edges of the road, tend to look blurred to the alcohol impaired drivers.*

Figure 5.1.[4] *How alcohol impaired driving affects vision.*

Testing of Edge Lines as an Alcohol-Related Crash Countermeasure

Considering the views of Professor Allen and others citing similar perspectives, the Potters Industries research and marketing groups began wondering if center lines and edge lines were prime alcohol-related crash countermeasures. This became timely when alcohol-related driving issues were in the forefront with the formation of Mothers Against Drunk Driving and the Presidential Commission on Drunk Driving in the early 1980s. Did reflectorized center lines and edge lines keep alcohol-impaired drivers on the road and in their lanes? Maybe edge lines were already an effective countermeasure, but could they be improved by using the wider 20 cm (8 inch) lines often used in Western Europe, rather than the narrower 10 cm (4 inch) lines used in the United States?

The big question was how to test this concept. To prove alcohol-impaired drivers respond to edge lines, or varying widths thereof, it seemed necessary to put alcohol-impaired drivers into such conditions on a road with similar unimpaired drivers. Simulators were rejected as not sensitive enough to the variables being studied. Could a test track be used? Maybe. But conducting the test on a real road with a typical roadside would be more convincing. Potters Industries, under the direction of Gerry Balcar, co-author of this book, embarked on a test that has never been duplicated. It was expensive, but it was needed and it was revealing.

The goal was to measure the lateral (side-to-side) position of vehicles under different road and driver conditions. Some drivers would be impaired with controlled doses of alcohol. Other drivers would receive placebo doses, with no alcohol impairment. The roads would either have no edge lines or different widths of edge lines. Would the drivers drive in the center of the driving lane most of the time? Or how far would they vary going on or over the center line or on or over the edge line?

Lateral vehicle position, and the variability therefrom, are measurements that tell how well drivers are doing, associated clearly with crash rates. Separate research studies by Pennsylvania State University, the Federal Highway Administration and the State of Illinois showed a definitive relationship of vehicle lateral position and variability with actual crash rates on roads where lateral position was tested. So if wide edge lines, or any edge lines, improved the lateral positions or lateral variability of vehicles, then crash rates would be reduced.

During the multi-year tests of marking materials, retroreflectivity and crash reduction that Potters conducted in the 1970s in the township of West Milford, NJ, the township police department was much involved. The senior officers and others participated in the planning, helped conduct the evaluations, assisted with visitors, and provided safety and protection during installation of the test sections. A good relationship had developed with its long-term chief, James Breslin, and with Lieutenant James Dykstra, who would succeed him. Lieutenant John Way, in charge of the traffic division, kept detailed statistics of crashes and had excellent data from before the extensive updated pavement marking. Way took part in preparing and presenting a report to the Subcommittee on Investigations and Oversight of the House Committee on Public Works and Transportation in Washington, DC.

Potters researchers asked the police department for a meeting about painting a test course with different edge-line widths and for drivers with different levels of inebriation to then drive the course. Essentially, they were asking the police to make the test possible by allowing alcohol-impaired drivers on their roads. Breslin and Dykstra offered to close the test roads from midnight to 3:00 A.M. The plan was that the test drivers would be operating dual controlled cars with a licensed driving instructor in the front seat. The

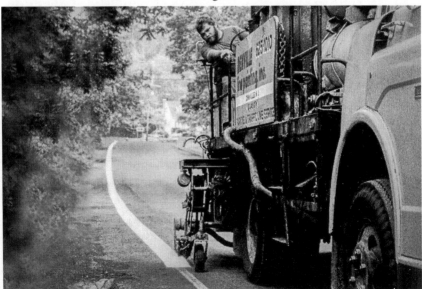

Figure 5.2.[5] *Preparing the test course road with wide edge lines.*

West Milford police stipulated this and that the test subjects not be dosed over the legal limit of blood alcohol content (BAC), which at the time was 0.1%. The subject drivers would not be allowed to see the officers manning the road closings. Little traffic was expected on Mondays through Thursdays at that time of night. A notice was sent by the police to all residents along the test course that they should call the police dispatcher should they need to leave their homes during the test. Any cars coming by would be held at the police barriers if a test driver was on the course, as were a few.

For test subjects, Potters consulted the Rutgers Center for Alcohol Studies at New Brunswick, NJ. Their suggestion was for a sample group of young men aged 21 to 25, the prime demographic group of the population most likely to be driving impaired. The Potters researchers asked if vision impairments would show up in subjects dosed to the still-legal levels of 0.05% and 0.08% BAC when compared to subjects not dosed. Rutgers personnel assured Potters they would be able to see the impairments in the results.

A query went to Farleigh Dickenson University in Teaneck, NJ asking if men of the required age group could be recruited for the test. The students would have to go to the test by bus so no one would be tempted to drive there and/or back impaired by alcohol or fatigue. The school also asked that there be a medical exam to make sure all could be safely dosed and could stay out until early morning. A medical group near the university campus did the physical examinations.

Potters arranged all of this. A 13-kilometer (8 mile) stretch of West Milford roads that previously had no edge lines were selected for the test course. The course was divided into 14 sections which were painted with 10, 15 and 20 cm (4, 6 and 8 inch) wide edge lines or left with no edge lines. None of the sections were less than 0.8 km (0.5 mile) long. A test headquarters was established at the West Milford High School, which was adjacent to the test track. The Rutgers Center for Alcohol Studies was retained to dose the subjects. A representative from their staff prepared and administered the drinks, basically vodka and tonic, formulated for each subject according to weight to raise their BAC level to 0.05% or

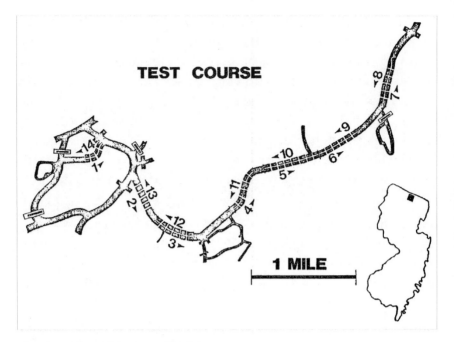

Figure 5.3.[6] *Map of the West Milford, NJ test course.*

0.08% or to keep them unimpaired with a non-alcoholic drink that smelled and tasted like the cocktail. The drinks were given at a time in advance of driving to be sure the right concentration would be in effect while driving the test course. The BAC level was verified by a breathalyzer test. Each subject drove the course twice on separate nights a week apart. The test subjects were divided into three groups. One group received the placebo drink for both trips. The others received the placebo drink for one trip and were dosed for the second trip to 0.05% or 0.08% BAC. The test was "double blind" as only the consultant from The Rutgers Center for Alcohol Studies knew who was dosed with alcohol.

The licensed New Jersey driving instructors supplied the dual-controlled cars. An instructor was in the right seat of each vehicle on each trip, able to intervene if necessary. The test drivers entered from the right door so as not to see the camera and the lights on the left side that illuminated the center line. They could not see these from the driver's position. The driving instructors helped rig the vehicles for the test, but otherwise were told very little about the purpose of the test and they knew little of the test course itself. In the rear seat were two Potters employees. One took a picture every 100 feet (36 meters) of the front wheel and the center line. The other timed the trip, which normally took 14 minutes, and monitored the test segments as they passed. The Potters employees did not speak during the test drives.

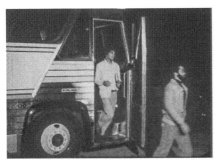

Figure 5.4.[7] *Test subjects arriving by bus.*

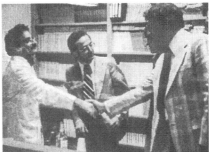

Figure 5.5.[8] *Dr. Rob Pantina of Rutgers University with project field director Nick Nedas and Potters' CMO Gerry Balcar.*

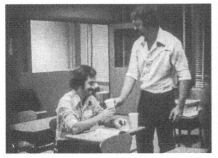

Figure 5.6.[9] *Placebo or actual vodka drinks are given out by a technician who does not know the contents of the drinks.*

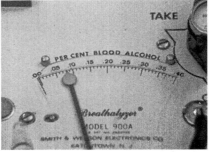

Figure 5.7.[10] *Breath test confirms a 0.08% BAC dose.*

There were over 9,200 total measurements of the vehicle positions recorded during the test drives. That equates to about 287 measurements per driver-trip and 21 measurements per test section per trip. All were tabulated for computer analysis. There were four fundamental results:[13]

Range of Driver Position was the range of the 70% of driving closest to the center of the lane plus the range of the next closest 10% on either side and the 5% farthest away from the center.

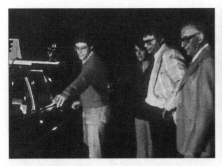 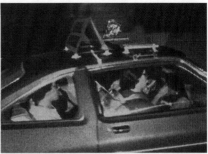

Figure 5.8.[11] *Preston Macy showing how the light array on the test car illuminates the lines on the road, which driver subjects did not see, to Lynn Galambossy, Gerry Balcar and Jim Ritter (all of Potters Industries).*   **Figure 5.9.**[12] *Test car with camera rigged on the roof of the car.*

Driver Variation is the variation of driver's vehicle positions from the center of the lane measured by the standard deviation.

Driver to driver grouping is a measure of how the drivers related to each other in mean positions. This indicates how the road was affecting the drivers in how they each saw the road. A tight grouping indicates they saw the road similarly. A wide grouping indicates more differences in their views of the road.

Mean Position is the accumulation of the mean positions of drivers in each test section.

Range of position is the part of measuring lateral position that tells when drivers get close to or stray over the center lines or edge lines. It is clear that the lines signal drivers in the process of potentially making a mistake that will lead to a crash. Often the lines prevent the crash. The graphs summarize the location where drivers put their vehicles in the lanes with different edge line conditions.

Where there were no edge lines, dosed (alcohol-impaired) drivers drove over the edge line position about 3% of the time. Un-dosed drivers did so a little less than 1% of the time. Dosed drivers drove over the 10 cm (4 inch) edge line about 2% of the time and fractionally over the 15 cm (6 inch) edge line. Un-dosed drivers did not go over any painted edge line. About 2% of the time they were on the 10 cm and 15 cm (4 and 6 inch) lines. Possibly 1% of their driving was on the 20 cm (8 inch) edge line. Dosed drivers drove on the 20 cm (8 inch) line about 3% of the time but did not drive over it.[14]

The result is interpreted to show the strength of the edge line visual signal. It appears drivers in the 20 cm (8 inch) wide line sections did significantly better than in sections with narrower or no edge lines.

The effect on lateral position of the drivers was also clear. The graph shows where the center 70% of driving was done and then the next 10% and 5% on each side. The best lateral positions were in the 20 cm (8 inch) edge line sections for both the dosed and undosed (placebo) drivers.

The variation shown by the drivers may explain this more succinctly.

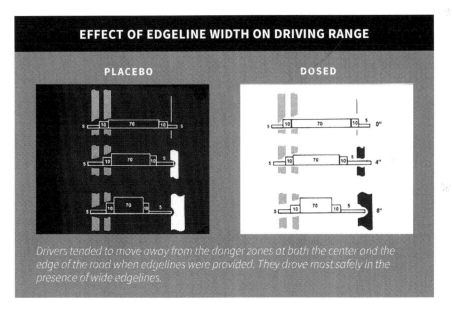

Figure 5.10.[15] *Effect of edge line width on driving range.*

Driver Variation is a measurement of how much drivers varied from the center of their lane. This is calculated from the standard deviations shown by drivers from the center in the different edge line sections. In the sections with no edge lines, the deviations of over four of the index of variability are significantly large. When edge lines are present, the deviations are mostly less than three.

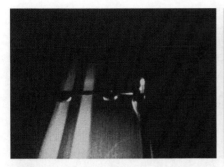 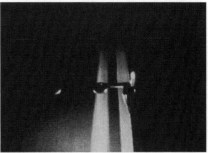

Figure 5.11.[16] *Showing lateral position in the center of the lane.*

Figure 5.12.[17] *Showing lateral position in the far left of the lane.*

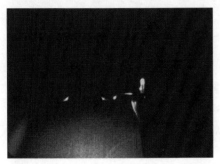

Figure 5.13.[18] *Showing lateral position in the far right of the lane.*

The drivers receiving the placebo drinks on both trips showed almost identical plotted results. The variation was mitigated significantly in the 10 cm (4 inch) edge lined sections. The plotted results of drivers who received alcohol dosed drinks are compared with their performance when they were not dosed. Their variation when they had only the placebo drink is much different than when they were dosed.

The drivers with a 0.05% BAC dose showed continued high variation in the 10 cm (4 inch) edge line sections which did not reduce until they were in a 15 cm (6 inch) edge line section.

The drivers with a 0.08% BAC dose showed reduced variation in the 10 cm (4 inch) edge line sections but much more compared to their placebo trips. For them, the 20 cm (8 inch) edge lines seemed to have more effect.[19]

Another presentation of the results of driver variability shows

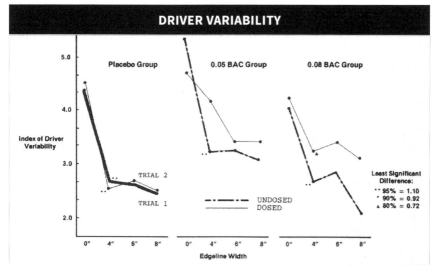

Figure 5.14.[20] *Driver Variability.*

the data in curves in figure 5.15. This presentation combines the dosed drivers. The strong response of those dosed to 0.08% BAC shows up.

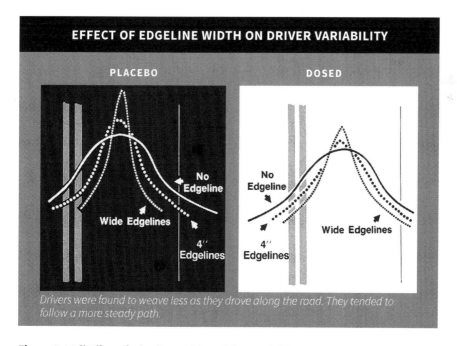

Figure 5.15.[21] *Effect of edge line width on driver variability.*

Driver Grouping uses the mean positions of drivers in each edge line section to evaluate the differences. This is done by creating groups for each, as in the graph. White over-laid swatches indicate un-dosed drivers. Grey swatches indicate alcohol dosed drivers.

Where there were no edge lines, both the un-dosed and the dosed drivers' plotted results were spread out and close to the road edge. With the test edge line widths, the grouping changed. With 10 cm (4 inch) edge lines, the un-dosed drivers tightened and moved toward the lane center. Dosed drivers moved away from the edge of the road but the plotted results were still spread out.

With 15 cm (6 inch) edge lines, both groups tightened and started to look alike except for their position in the lane. With 20 cm (8 inch) edge lines, there was more similarity.[23]

In the aggregate, these tests showed an alcohol effect and very much an edge line effect. The lateral position of the test drivers was improved by edge lines. It was further improved by adding edge-line width. The driver grouping shows that the drivers saw the road more clearly with wider edge lines.

Most important, when all of Potters' work on this study was done, the Federal Highway Administration asked for the 9,200 data measurements. They gave these to an independent research firm that verified that the findings were statistically significant. The Federal Highway Administration (FHWA) then announced two conclusions:

1. When drivers are un-dosed (with placebo), the presence of edge lines of any width resulted in more good driving than occurred without edge lines and,
2. When drivers were dosed with alcohol to 0.05% and 0.08% BAC levels, there was more good driving in the presence of wide edge lines than in the presence of standard 10 cm (4 inch) lines or no edge lines.

The test in West Milford of wide lines sparked much interest in the use of wider lines and the results thereof were published in The Transportation Research Record, Washington, DC. A flurry of tests appeared in the technical literature with review and survey articles. Many states responded to the FHWA, if not to the research results

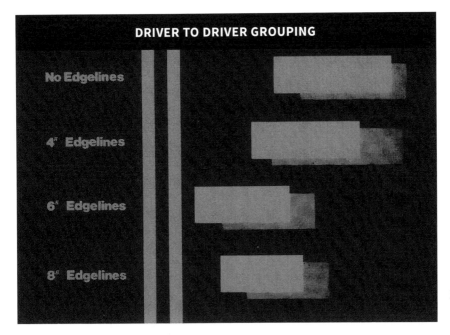

Figure 5.16.[22] *Driver to driver grouping.*

from West Milford. Later, the European Commission, the executive authority for the European Union and therefore the European Parliament, undertook a major study into the brightness of retroreflection required for pavement markings to function properly.

The European Commission – COST 331[24]

The European Commission became involved in pavement marking starting in 1995 with a large and expensive study. The report of the work labeled COST 331 – Requirements for Horizontal Road Marking, was produced by the Directorate General for Transport under the Directorate General for Research within the program of Cooperation on Science and Technology (COST).

The COST 331 report did not set out to prove the value of reflectorized pavement marking as a tool to improve road safety. Instead, the study started with the premise that reflectorized pavement marking already was a proven tool and based on that premise, COST 331 set out to "…establish an up-to-date scientific method with which, on the basis of drivers' visual needs, to determine the optimal pavement marking design in order to ensure that it is visible, by day and by night, in all weather conditions."

Restated, the views of traffic experts from the then (1999) 15 member countries of the European Union who participated in producing COST 331 from 1995 to 1999 took as a fact that pavement marking is a proven tool to improve road safety. Their quest was to improve on this tool to find its optimal design and that, "…establishing the 'state of the art' in the field of road marking is a necessary first step in the preparation of strategies to achieve convergence in the current differences in road safety in different European countries."

It is not fully understood how uniformity affects road safety, but it is certainly conceivable that the lack of uniformity might cause crashes when drivers are confronted with markings they do not immediately understand. The United States had trouble establishing uniformity within 48 contiguous states in the same country. The European Commission had 15, and now has 28, sovereign nations. To go around the political difficulties in establishing uniformity in pavement marking, perhaps the scientific back door would open up some opportunities. In retrospect, even though COST 331 provided a step forward in developing standards for road markings and for understanding driver response times, uniformity of road markings in Europe has not yet been achieved.

As stated in the introduction to COST 331, road traffic crashes and deaths cause a huge economic loss from medical expenses, police and emergency services, damage to property and lost economic output, not to mention unmeasurable human suffering. This has led to a "…growing acceptance that a wide range of strategies is needed to address the problem. *The traffic system has to adapt to the needs, mistakes and vulnerabilities of road users rather than the other way around.*"

Further in the introduction, it is also stated:

> "Later trends in road safety look, more and more, towards *Low Cost Road Engineering Measures* (LCM), such as minor changes in junction operation, road lay-out, lighting, signs and markings which can be implemented quickly and make significant contributions to road safety. Within the above mentioned set of LCM,

those concerning road signing in general (and in particular, road markings), have been traditionally considered interesting alternatives to improve road safety. Unfortunately, this potential benefit – and well proven effectiveness – of road markings is not sufficiently exploited by the relevant decision makers."

This statement is, unfortunately, also a comment on the failure of officials in Western Europe to recognize the importance of road markings as a road traffic crash countermeasure. The same can be said about officials in the United States.

In one main action of a test conducted for COST 331, subjects were evaluated in a simulator to determine aspects of visual needs. In the simulator, a drive of 5 km (3.1 miles) could be conducted at different sight distances viewing road marking lines of established brightness. Subjects drove through different sight distances at a speed they selected. A large number of vision evaluations were recorded.

In separate field work, the brightness of headlights were matched with retroreflective responses from markings. Visibility responses were established at 3 to 5 seconds. The desirable visibility and the needed response times serve to indicate when markings should be renewed. This issue was raised by COST 331 in order to keep the markings performing at optimal levels.

The COST 331 researchers also tested drivers in real road conditions for lateral position in varying edge line conditions. The test was unique in that the subjects drove the roads in Portugal, Switzerland and Finland at night without markings and then after markings with differing edge line widths were installed. The same pattern of edge line widths was installed in each test country.

The subjects were not dosed with vodka as those in the West Milford test were, but varied in age. The results sustained the findings reported in West Milford, except that a 30 cm (12 inch) wide line was also tested. That width was preferred by drivers and produced the most results of moving the lateral position favorably toward the center of the driving lane.

Cost 331 breaks new ground in evaluating the retroreflectivity of road markings. It confirms the value of lines wider than 10 cm

(4 inches) and promotes widths of 20 cm (8 inches) and wider. It also adds:

> "The conclusions show that there is a need to establish a national policy (taking account of driver age, headlamp intensity and glare from opposing traffic and climate) for road marking design, due to their influence on road safety."

The main contributions of COST 331 is that it specifies optimal retroreflectivity values for road marking installations and it supports the general findings of using wide lines on roads. It also promotes uniformity in road marking operations. In concluding the report however, maybe this statement from the report's authors is the most valuable from a policy and decision making perspective:

> "…to encourage road authorities and other relevant decision makers to accord to road markings the role they deserve as one of the most effective (i.e. with one of the highest cost-benefit ratios) low cost engineering measures available for improving road safety."

What is most surprising with COST 331 is that the knowledge contained therein, primarily that road marking is a proven, effective and cost beneficial road crash countermeasure, has gotten lost in the debate for reducing traffic tragedy in low- and middle-income countries. This is a question that needs to be immediately addressed.

The Use of Wider Markings

The wider edge line, alcohol-impaired driver research in West Milford, NJ and the use of wider lines – wider than 10 cm (4 inch) – in Western Europe set off a flurry of tests in America. These reflected on the interest in the concept of increasing the visual signal from pavement markings. A large number of crash reduction tests of wider lines by state departments of transportation and their highway departments, and others took place. The extensive and expensive COST 331 in Europe set some visual standards for marking retroreflectivity. It also favored wide edge lines of 20 cm (8 inch) and opened up the possibility for 30 cm (12 inch) lines. In 2002, with a follow-on in 2012, the Texas Transportation Institute at Texas A&M University reported on the use of, and reasons for, wider lines in North America and Europe.

The authors of the first report (2002) were Timothy J. Gates, Assistant Transportation Researcher, and H. Gene Hawkins, PhD, PE, Division Head, at the institute in College Station, Texas.[25] They conducted two surveys among transportation agencies regarding the use and benefits of wider lines in the United States, Canada and other countries, also reviewing the technical literature about wider markings.

A total of 29 different state highway departments in the USA affirmed they were installing wider lines to some degree on their roads. Most of these were 15 cm (6 inch) wide. Greater marking visibility was the most cited (57% of respondents) reason for installing wider lines. The special needs of older drivers for increased retroreflectivity and contrast to compensate for declining visual and cognitive capabilities was another reason. Favorable public response was also noted as a reason to install wider markings, as were crash reduction, driver comfort, conformance with other transportation agencies, road marking service life improvement and as a driver fatigue countermeasure.[26]

The main downside cited for using wider markings was increased cost. Highway departments that did not use wider makings commonly indicated their use would be considered if conclusive evidence of their effectiveness justified the extra cost.

In reporting on the results of multiple crash reduction tests of wider lines, the results did not support the popular views as emphatically as in the classic tests of comparing edge lines with no lines. Most tests were before and after tests on the same road. Separate studies by New Mexico and Virginia DOTs found that 20 cm (8 inch) edge lines did not produce statistically significant run-off-the-road crash reductions compared to standard 10 cm (4 inch) edge lines. Studies of available crash data from Ohio, Maine and Texas indicated 20 cm (8 inch) edge lines were not more effective than 10 cm (4 inch) edge lines. At two specific installations, 25 cm (10 inch) lines yielded no conclusive improvement in crash results in Maryland. The Kansas DOT found no significant change in crashes in a test they performed. Maine found the same. Texas installed a 320 km (200 mile) test with no significant run-off-the-road crash prevention improvements. North Carolina and Oklahoma had similar results.[27]

The results concerning the effectiveness of wider lines, however, were not all inconclusive. Some crash studies have produced data to support the increased effectiveness of wider lines versus the use of 10 cm (4 inch) lines. The FHWA researchers found a decrease in fatalities on 480 km (300 miles) of rural two-lane road in Alabama with a high average daily traffic count when a 20 cm (8 inch) wide edge line replaced a 10 cm (4 inch) line. In South Dakota, a similar test showed positive results. The Montana DOT, working in an older driver corridor, found 20 cm (8 inch) wide lines reduced crashes by older drivers by 18% and by all drivers by 8%. In a three year test in New Jersey, fatal and injury crashes decreased 16% after safety improvements of adding wide lines in Morris County. Crashes on roads with 20 cm (8 inch) lines decreased 16% while a decrease of 8% was recorded on roads with 10 cm (4 inch) lines.[28]

Gates and Hawkins determined that two schools of thought exist when considering the effectiveness of wider vs. 10 cm (4 inch) pavement markings:[29]

1. "The effectiveness of wider markings as a highway safety improvement cannot be justified without some form of conclusive cost-quantifiable data to support this claim, such as crash reductions."

2. "Recognizing that conclusive cost-quantifiable data are likely not available and would be extremely difficult to measure, other proven measures of effectiveness are appropriate to justify the use of wider markings because such measures *imply* improved safety, and thus serve as a proxy for crash reductions."

Results from the survey of transportation agencies indicated that the latter school of thought is preferred:[30]

Further, the writers summed up this description of driver delineation needs:[31]

"In a general sense, the ability of a driver to safely operate a vehicle is based on the driver's perception of a situation, level of alertness, the amount of information available, and the driver's information assimilation capabilities. Although the transportation profession can do little to control a driver's level of alertness or information-processing capabilities, the presentation of information can be designed for in the form of traffic control devices, including pavement markings. To be effective, pavement markings must:

- present the appropriate visual clues far enough in advance of a given situation to allow for suitable reaction time to occur, and
- be visible in the periphery to aid in moment-to-moment lane navigation.

This is especially true at night when the visibility of the roadway and surrounding features drops dramatically, causing motorists to rely heavily on pavement marking retroreflection for delineation cues. While many factors are involved in long-distance and peripheral detection of markings, the retroreflectivity and width of markings are two variables that can be engineered by transportation agencies and have been shown in the literature to influence marking visibility."

The second report (2012) was written by Paul Carlson, PhD, PE, Division Head, Operations and Roadway Safety Division, and Jason Wagner, Associate Transportation Researcher.[32] Analyzing a large amount of data from three states (Kansas, Michigan and Illinois) and using three separate statistical measures, the research provided strong evidence that wider edge lines are a cost-effective crash countermeasure on two-lane rural roads. This conclusive data paves the way for further use of wider lines by transportation agencies that were reluctant to install them without first having the data to support this claim.

The authors of this report further state that "Wider edge lines have been shown to reduce total crashes 15 to 30 percent, and fatal plus injury crashes 15 to 38 percent. In addition, the benefit-cost ratio for wide edge lines is $33 to $55 for each $1 spent."[33]

Report on the Pavement Marking Demonstration Program

Dr. Carlson with other colleagues, Dr. Eun Sug Park of TTI and Carl Anderson of the FHWA, brought out another review paper in 2008.[34] This included the results from the Pavement Marking Demonstration Program enacted in 1973 in the United States. Thirty-eight states participated and many submitted positive findings. Only data from six states made the cut of acceptance into the Texas Transportation Institute report, as the researchers found this data to be robust enough for further analysis.

The paper's authors reviewed 225 sites described in the reports. These were on two-lane road sections of at least 8 km (5 miles) in length and with road widths over 5 meters (16 feet). The speed limit had to be at least 65km/h (40 mph). The only safety improvement allowed was the installation of center lines and edge lines, or edge lines only if there were a center line already installed. The reported results were:[35]

- Overall there was a 12% decrease in nighttime crashes and a 33% decrease in crashes with low-visibility nighttime conditions.
- On roads seven meters wide (22 feet), there was a 36% reduction in nighttime crashes and a 52% reduction in crashes with low-visibility nighttime conditions. It is likely that the speeds on seven meter roads (22 feet) were faster than on roads narrower than six meters (19 feet).

The Institute of Transport Economics

Perhaps the report with the widest grasp of road safety measures has been published by the Institute of Transport Economics in Oslo, Norway. This organization produces the *Handbook of Road Safety Measures* funded through the Norwegian Ministry of Transportation and Communication and the Norwegian Public Roads Administration.[36] The aim of the manual is to provide easily accessible information on how to prevent traffic injury. This large volume examines the science and mathematics behind road safety issues, practices and countermeasures, and is fully international in scope.

The section on road markings in the 2009 edition reports on 55 tests done in various countries, describing a meta-analysis program used to evaluate them. The summary shows that when the combination of center lines and edge lines are added to roads, total crashes were reduced by 24%, a significant drop.[37]

Since the classic road marking tests, and during and after the American success with marking rural roads, further tests have been done and reviews have been written, consolidating some of the research in the United States and elsewhere. What is missing though is the action to emphasize the core importance of markings in any new crash reduction effort. This is especially the case in efforts in low- and middle-income countries.

6

Road Marking Operations and Priorities

Prior chapters about the early demand by motorists for lines on the roads, the classic tests, the emergence of road safety engineering and the results of maximizing the safety of existing roads embody the background to everyday action on roads in the rich world. Installing and maintaining reflectorized pavement markings on urban and rural roads is an effective traffic control and a frontline means of crash reduction. On rural two-lane roads, center lines and edge lines are indispensable as a countermeasure to traffic tragedy. Road traffic crashes that were prevented when pavement markings were initially installed are still being prevented as long as the markings are maintained.

Regrettably, the important role road markings serve in reducing road traffic crashes is overlooked in traffic manuals around the world. In the latest version (2009 edition with revisions one and two in 2012) of the United States' Manual on Uniform Traffic Control Devices (MUTCD), this introduction paragraph to the segment on markings demonstrates not only the incomplete thinking in the United States, but also in much of the rich world:[1]

> "Markings on highways and on private roads open to public travel have important functions in providing guidance and information for the road user. Major marking types include pavement and curb markings, delineators, colored pavements, channelizing devices, and islands. In some cases, markings are used to supplement other traffic control devices such as signs, signals, and other markings. In other instances, markings are used alone to effectively convey regulations, guidance, or warnings in ways not obtainable by the use of other devices."

In reality, those who load, drive and operate the marking machines, those providing the administrative support and those who plan and budget projects, are all engaged in much more than simply installing guidance devices for road users. They are engaged in saving lives and injuries. Much goes on behind the action of installing and renewing road markings. The quality must be assured and the renewals must be timely to make sure the retroreflectivity benefits of the markings are operational or they cease to provide the critical element of crash prevention.

Marking Equipment and Materials

In the very early days of road marking, the cost of painting road markings was high. Much direct labor was needed using brushes and templates. Fortunately, the means to automate were already at hand. When the mechanical air compressor was introduced in the 1870s, an early application for it was paint spraying. It was used mainly in shipyards, but it was such a productivity enhancer that other applications soon followed. Those responsible for painting lines on roads realized that a spray device would be the way forward.

The first machines adopted for marking roads were small and hand-operated, with operators walking. To suit these devices, or if work was done by hand, early protocols limited recommendations for center lines to curves and hills. The machines soon advanced in size and capability. Modern striping trucks have nozzles on both sides capable of adding or renewing center lines with passing zones and an edge line simultaneously.

Glass beads, about the size of typical sugar grains, are made from high quality waste soda lime glass, and are the essential retroreflective elements in pavement marking. The beads make road markings brightly visible at night when headlights from a vehicle shine on them.

Traffic marking paint is a high-solids type of paint, the better for resisting traffic wear. It has strong adhesive qualities to hold glass beads dropped on it immediately following the spray application. This paint is quick drying to mitigate tracking by cars running over fresh lines. Originally, the paint was solvent-based, but is now mostly water-based to avoid hydrocarbon pollution. The width of lines, the paint thickness and the bead drop onto the line is computer controlled to the speed of the striping truck. With these computerized flows of paint and beads, traffic lines should be of consistent high quality. Most are.

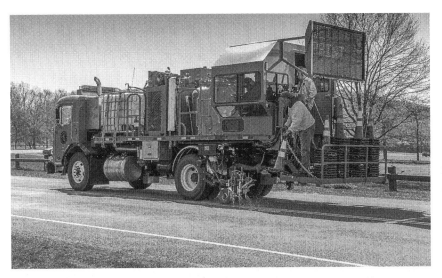

Figure 6.1. *A customized modern paint striping truck. Photo © by Rob Bowman. Use by permission M-B Companies, Inc.*

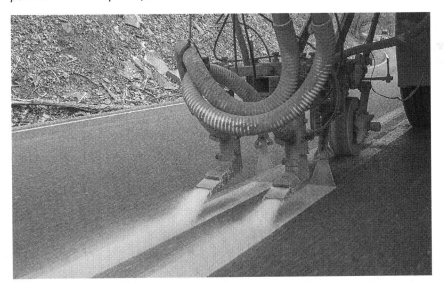

Figure 6.2. *Application of paint and glass beads by a striping truck. Photo use by permission Potters Industries, LLC.*

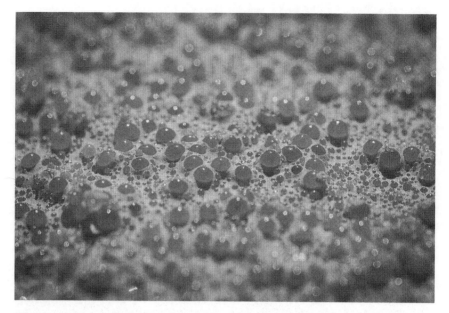

Figure 6.3. *Macro photograph of glass beads in paint. Photo use by permission Potters Industries, LLC.*

More durable lines, with a longer service life, were needed in cities and on high-traffic roads. Thermoplastic lines are more expensive, but serve this durability purpose in urban areas and where wear is heavy. Thermoplastic is applied hot to enhance binding to road surfaces. Glass beads are dropped on as well as premixed into the binder for the lines to stay retroreflective even as the binder wears. Specially designed striping trucks normally install thermoplastic lines without the need for lane closures.

Many jurisdictions now use preformed lines and shapes like arrows and message markings. These are applied to roads with heat or adhesive. Beads are premixed in the resin and are also dropped on during installation. Further to the durability and the service life of the marking, added advantages of this process are no paint drying time and less time needed for application. This reduces lane closure time if any is needed. Epoxy, a cold plastic, is another more durable binder than paint. It offers good bead retention and a high measure of retroreflectivity. Being a two-system material, with a basic resin and a hardener, it is more difficult to install, but, like thermoplastic, it has a longer useful life.

ROAD MARKING OPERATIONS AND PRIORITIES 93

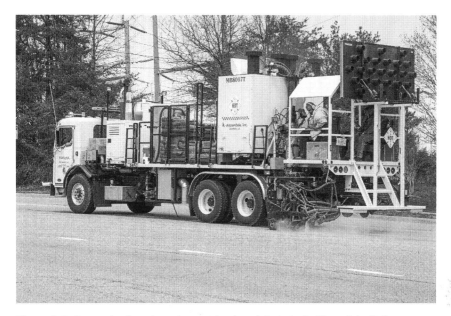

Figure 6.4. *Customized modern thermoplastic striping truck. Photo © by Rob Bowman. Use by permission M-B Companies, Inc.*

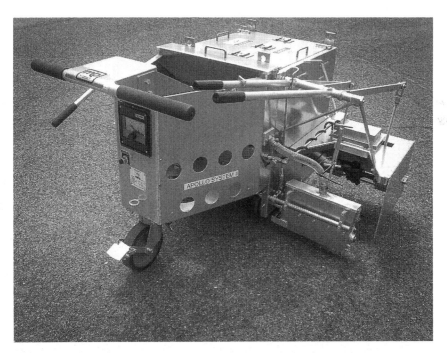

Figure 6.5. *Modern thermoplastic hand liner. Photo use by permission M-B Companies, Inc.*

The importance of pavement markings is emphasized even more by requirements needed when installing temporary markings in construction and other zones. This is usually done by using special retroreflective tape. When the road surface is ready for permanent markings, the tape is removed without damaging the road surface.

Raised Pavement Markers and Wet Weather

The first raised pavement markers were developed in Britain during the early months of World War II to assist drivers during blackouts. These used "cats eye" reflectors or large glass spheres up to 1.25 cm (a half inch) in diameter. Enclosed in small rubber housings mounted in a rubber bladder on a ceramic base, they were inserted in hollowed out segments in the road center and cemented in place. Even with limited headlight, they were visible in normal weather and light conditions and had the extra benefit of also being visible in rain. Some were designed so that if a car went over them with water on the road, the face of the glass would be wiped clean of any dirt. Their use was almost entirely in England, known for narrow roads and rainy conditions. They came to be called "British road studs."

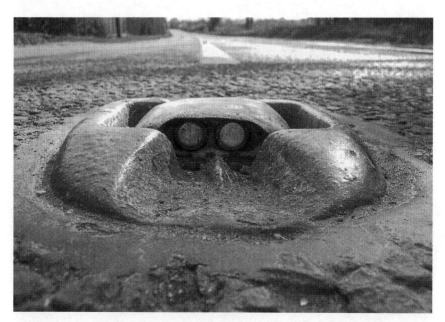

Figure 6.6.[2] *A "cat's eye" raised pavement marker in the United Kingdom. The reflective spheres are shown set into the road stud.*

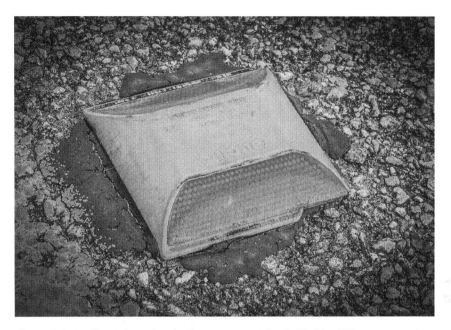

Figure 6.7. *A yellow prismatic raised pavement marker in Florida, USA. Photo by Amie Brockway.*

In the next phase of advancement, prismatic reflectors attached to a ceramic or other housing were introduced. Epoxied to road centers and edges, these work well in rain and were self-cleaning. Mostly they were used in warm climates. In areas where snow plowing occurs frequently in winter, as in the Northeast and Mid west of the United States, Canada, northern and interior Europe and Asia, snowplows scraping to bare pavement often pop them up and remove them together with the snow. Though considerably more expensive, snowplow-resistant, raised prismatic markers were also developed. These were in a steel housing designed to allow plows to pass over them, being imbedded in the pavement with a strong binder.

One concern regarding raised pavement markers is durability. They are subject to extra wear from heavy vehicles like 40-ton 18-wheelers. The durability has improved, but their use in areas where snow is frequent is limited.

A second concern was to install enough of them to make a peripheral signal that would not attract foveal (center-eye) vision

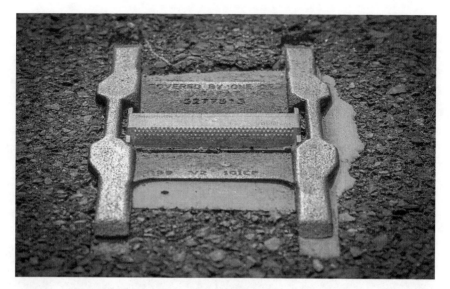

Figure 6.8. *A yellow prismatic raised pavement marker in a snow-plowable steel housing in New Jersey, USA. Photo by Bo Elfving.*

time. Combinations of center lines and edge lines with raised pavement markers have been designed and used, especially when there is a need for additional retroreflectivity in rainy road conditions. To provide continuous visible lines on rainy nights, special glass beads

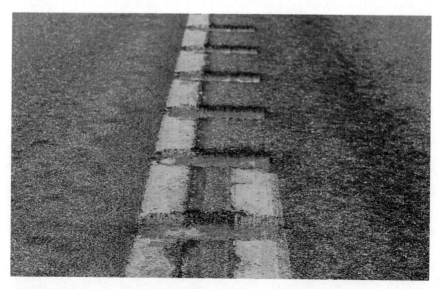

Figure 6.9. *A center rumble strip on a two-lane rural road overpainted with a reflectorized center line. Photo by Bo Elfving.*

have also been developed. Somewhat larger than the beads typically used, they make paint lines and the more durable thermoplastic, epoxy and other such systems, retroreflect better in wet weather.

The use of raised pavement markers led to another safety concept. When drivers occasionally drove over the markers, alongside reflectorized center lines and edge lines, they experienced vibration and noise. This led to the development of a warning system of "rumble strips." Tests have shown that the vibration and audible noise from crossing over the rumble strip will gain the attention of drowsy or otherwise inattentive drivers to help keep them on the road and in the correct driving lane.[3]

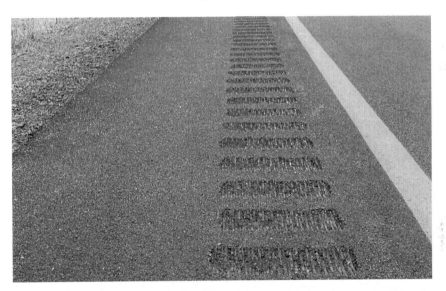

Figure 6.10. *An edge-line rumble strip on the left side of a divided highway. A rumble strip is also installed outside the edge line on the right of the highway. Photo by Bo Elfving.*

Pavement Marking Operations

Installing or renewing road markings is a specialized field that involves teamwork and logistics. A good day's work will see 40 to 50 kilometers (24 to 30 miles) of 15-centimeter (6-inch) center lines and edge lines installed on two-lane roads. This requires about 13,600 kg (30,000 lbs.) of paint and 6,800 kg (15,000 lbs.) of glass beads, and usually a second truck to carry extra material. If productivity can be extended on long, warm-weather days, yet another truck may be needed to keep the one doing the spraying supplied. An additional truck may have to carry work-in-progress or work-zone warning signs with personnel to place and retrieve them.

Surveying for passing zones is done according to government regulations. Sight distances are determined and associated with time or distance needed to return to the driving lane from a passing maneuver according to published instructions. When the zones are established, codes indicating the painting pattern to be applied are marked on the pavement or attached as small signs to delineators or other posts along the roadside. The solid and dashed lines of the passing zones are applied by an operator on the truck using electronic photo sensitive controls of paint and bead flow that start and stop painting the dashed lines.

Where possible, an outbound application of center lines and an edge line is followed by a return trip painting only a second edge line, from and to a base. Striping crews often work at temporary bases where they are supplied from a home base or directly from vendors. Lines are installed by striping contractors providing the service to governments by bid or by government employee road-marking crews.

Effective life of the pavement markings is the key value of crash countermeasure. The technology used to determine the effective life of markings is retroreflectometer measurement of lines and the brightness of their response to vehicle headlights. This has been engineered so that continuous readings in daylight can measure the effectiveness the lines will have in nighttime conditions. Instruments can be handheld for spot measurements, but are mainly mounted on a vehicle, with complete retroreflectivity measurements collected driving alongside the lines. The instruments indicate the lines to be either: (1) good or still sufficiently retroreflective; (2) to be marginal and in need of renewal soon; or (3) that they are worn out and should be renewed immediately as they have lost their retroreflectivity qualities.

Traffic is the constant wear on markings, average daily traffic (ADT) being the gauge of wear. It is winter weather, however, with snow plowing, and snow and ice treatments, that cause the most harm. The lines are scraped down and the beads are scraped off. Good painted lines will stay minimally in service after a winter season, but will usually need renewal.

More durable binders have different life profiles in winter weather conditions. In most thermoplastic applications, in addition to the normal drop-on application of glass beads at installation, premixed beads in the binder become visible as the lines are worn. Premixed paint with glass beads can likewise be used to prolong the effective life of lines or to assure getting through the winter season with sufficient retroreflectivity left in the lines. After a winter season, lines may appear as though they are adequate in daylight but may not be sufficiently retroreflective at night.

Where there is little snow and light traffic, painted lines may last three years before needing renewal. In the tropics or warm temperate zones with hot summers, a good quality traffic paint and quality glass beads will stand up well. Under heavy traffic in these climates, epoxy may be the choice, particularly for urban markings. Both paint and thermoplastic are vulnerable to heat and ultra-violet ray damage.

In both the United States and Western Europe, studies have set forth standards of retroreflection needed for normal response by drivers. The European Commission spent a lot of money on determining this, as indicated in their publication COST 331 (see Chapter 5).[4] This report is highly regarded, although the overly complex presentation makes it difficult to read for laypersons and especially for those in a decision-making capacity who need the information the most. Despite the availability of information, the United States and Western Europe do not fully use optimal standards for retroreflectivity. Striping contractors resist guaranteeing a minimum limit of retroreflection that must be present after wear. The Federal Highway Administration in the United States is also not insisting on such minimum limits of retroreflectivity.

Renewal of Pavement Markings

The critical and mostly unrecognized issue in renewing pavement markings is the absence of a historic understanding that center lines and edge lines are primary road crash countermeasures. Some jurisdictions allow lines to wear down to the extent that they lose their retroreflectivity and hence are of no value. Such inaction allows an increase in traffic crashes. The reality that the lines are not just for guidance must reach decision-makers responsible for allocating sufficient budgets for their installation and maintenance. Likewise, the fact that the lines are installed and maintained in order to prevent drivers from making mistakes, and for them to avoid getting into crashes, also needs to reach the same decision-makers and communicated to the public.

Doing everything reasonably possible to reduce crashes should be the first order of any highway department. In this regard, there is a need to focus on the crash reduction aspects of pavement markings and in particular on center lines and edge lines. When it comes to road maintenance and budgeting, the first and most important matter should be to renew center lines and edge lines. To allow the effectiveness of the lines to diminish is to cause crashes that otherwise might be prevented.

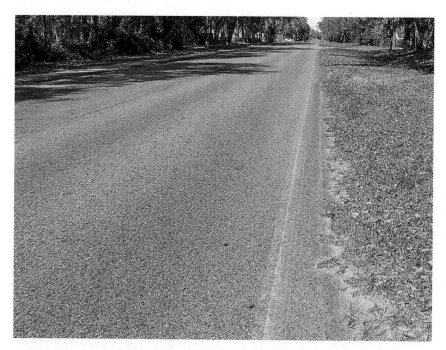

Figure 6.11. *Very worn white edge line. Photo by Amie Brockway.*

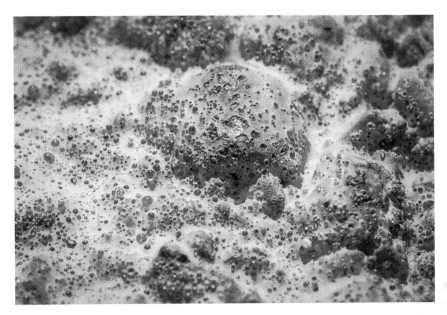

Figure 6.12. *Macro photograph of worn glass beads in paint. Photo use by permission Potters Industries, LLC.*

Developing Road Marking Standards

When the first pavement markings were installed in the USA, states, counties and even cities had the freedom to design their own patterns. Some variances in urban marking may still be seen. As late as 1971, some state highway departments still thought they had special and unique requirements in their road marking needs. The greater contrast of white versus yellow lines was one center of controversy. An international debate is still going on about that.

The US Federal Highway Administration (FHWA), however, sternly sought uniformity in markings. The agency further said that yellow lines indicating opposite direction traffic were more important than the minor variance in perceived contrast compared to white lines. In the United States, the Manual on Uniform Traffic Control Devices (MUTCD) of 1971 mandated uniformity for much that was painted or installed on pavements. The first MUTCD issued by the FHWA, it bore the full authority of the US Department of Transportation. All-yellow center lines were established. The all-white center lines with passing zones, and the single solid-white center line faded into memory in the United States. Most present-day American drivers have never seen them. They may be encountered for the first time when traveling abroad.

The MUTCD, to all appearances a listing of requirements to assure the safest possible travel for the driving public, leaves some wide gaps with respect to road markings. It does dictate that center lines on roads separating opposite direction traffic shall be yellow. However, it requires only that the lines be placed on two-lane roads six meters (20 feet) wide or wider with an Average Daily Traffic (ADT) of 6,000 vehicles or more. This is further clarified with a mention that center lines *should* be placed on, but is not *required* on, roads with an ADT of 4,000 vehicles. Regarding edge lines, the dictum is that they are required on two-lane roads that are six meters (20 feet) wide or wider and with an ADT of 6,000 vehicles. The qualifying advisory calls for edge lines on roads with the same width and an ADT of 3,000 vehicles and for lines to be 10 to 15 cm (4 to 8 inch) wide.[5]

This is far short of what is needed by the American experience and by many of the tests of edge lines or the combination of center lines and edge lines on rural roads. The spectacular results of crash, injury and death reduction in tests and in real experience on American rural two-lane arterials and collector roads were almost entirely on roads with ADTs of less than 3,000 vehicles, most having ADTs of less than 2,000.

What often happen is that the individual states lobby during the review or comment period on proposed federal regulations to reduce the requirements stipulated in the MUTCD or other regulations. Every rule- or regulation-making by executive agencies required by legislation from Congress has a long comment period. One purpose is for the agencies involved, the Department of Transportation and the FHWA in the case of highway laws, to organize in order to enforce or provide the intended provisions with the details. A second reason is for those affected by the law to respond to it if they consider it burdensome.

Saturating downtown Washington, DC are offices of law firms and lobbyists prepared to do just that, to respond. Most national trade or business associations are also headquartered right in DC or nearby. Their location allows the leaders and staffs of these organizations to be intimately involved in any legislative or regulatory issue. There are more than a thousand such groups. At 444 North Capitol Street there is a large building that houses many representatives of state governments. Another tenant is the American Association of State Highway and Transportation Officials (AASHTO).

AASHTO itself began a safety emphasis program in 2004 when research disclosed that in 2003 more than 40% of fatal crashes resulted from vehicles deviating from the proper lane. On rural roads, that number was even higher, at two-thirds. The program therefore aimed at keeping drivers in their lanes, calling for center lines and edge lines on all major roads and minor roads with histories of crashes.[6]

Some states appear to try to reduce the amount of marking they must do. They know the driving public, represented by associations like the American Automobile Association (AAA), will insist on roads with high quality markings. They know they will not get away with much reduction, but they want to keep the federal requirements loose so they can avoid marking if they choose. There are also states that would not even think of denying or limiting road marking on any state highway or road under their control.

Lobbyists in the United States have watered down the requirements in the MUTCD. The essential reason for installing center lines and edge lines, to serve as a prime crash countermeasure, is missing in the MUTCD language. This needs to be corrected in the next version of the manual. The wording also needs to be changed to reflect the results of the rural road-marking program of 1973. The requirement should be to install center lines and edge lines on all sufficiently wide roads with an ADT of 1,000 vehicles or more. Similar language and requirements in traffic manuals in nations around the world would help improve their road traffic safety efforts. By failing to ascribe the essential life-saving characteristic to pavement markings, traffic manuals are steering advisors, planners and decision makers worldwide astray.

Pedestrians and Cyclists

For an observant visitor to low- or middle-income countries, a first impression might include noticing the number of people who walk everywhere to work, to carry out household errands, to recreation, to community activities, or to their church, mosque or temple. It is a reasonable generality to say that where the GDP per capita is less than US $2,000, there are a lot of people walking.

Those walking on the roadside can be difficult to see in darkness. Putting reflectors on clothing helps, but that is far from enough. A first and important step is to create a separation between vehicular traffic and pedestrians. Installing edge lines creates a basic separation. They make clear where foot and wheeled traffic go. This is critically important where vehicle speeds are faster than 50 km/hr (30 mph). One of the mistakes edge lines help avoid is drivers not seeing the edge of the road and therefore striking pedestrians walking there.

Additional means of separation like foot paths, sidewalks, and outright barriers are ultimately desirable. So are lanes for bicycles, mopeds and motorcycles. The first step though should always be to install reflectorized lines. This is consistent with the long-held principle of separation of traffic in road safety. The traffic control and operations manuals of the rich world call for marking intersections, turn lanes, crosswalks, gore areas (where roads merge or split) and entrance and exit lanes. Good work has been done nearly everywhere in marking pavements at pedestrian crossings. Advance warnings of crosswalks have also been implemented.

There are also recent developments in using specialized lanes. Those for bicycles started in Europe, where cycling for exercise and transport took off early. In Copenhagen, a very flat city, the major vehicle arteries have separate lanes for bikes. Amsterdam claims to be the biking capital of Europe, a reported 40% of its traffic said to be bicycles. Berlin, Seville and Malmö are some among many other cities that are bike-friendly, with separate lanes and paths.

In America, the MUTCD indicates there may be lanes set aside for bikes outside the edge line. When installed, most of these bike

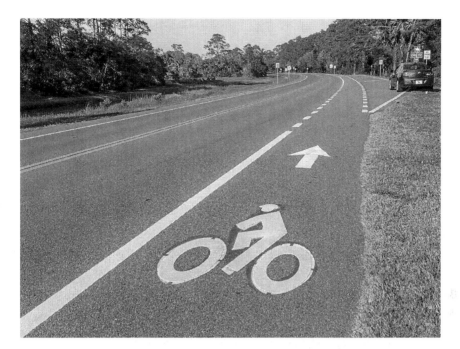

Figure 6.13. *Suburban bike lane separated by the edge line. Photo by Amie Brockway.*

lanes are in urban settings. Among the leading bike-friendly cities are Minneapolis, Portland, Boulder, Seattle, San Francisco, Washington DC, and New York.

In dealing with road tragedy evidenced in many low- and middle-income nations, separation of traffic is an important crash countermeasure tool. When separation is accomplished with pavement marking, it is combined with positive guidance to drivers by center lines and edge lines. The edge line may be an adequate channelizing means for pedestrians on rural roads. While crash prevention is always the main reason for installing center lines and edge lines, crash prevention is even more important for two-wheeled traffic. Of two-wheeled crashes, a much larger percentage results in injury.

New ideas and concepts specific to low- and middle-income countries are needed. The concepts must be adapted to the needs of many nations with multiple characteristics, such as varying traffic composition (bicycles, mopeds, motorcycles and vehicles of different types) and, most importantly, of varying resources.

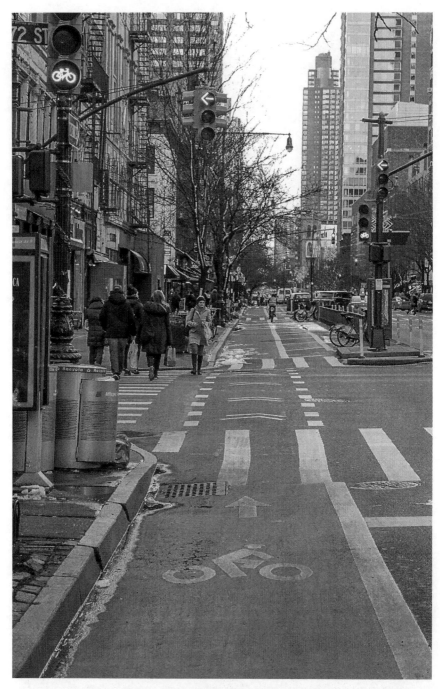

Figure 6.14. Urban bike lane. Columbus Ave. at W. 72nd St. in New York City. Note the specific green light for the bike lane road users and the Citi Bike bike-share system bikes and docking stations in the background. Photo by Bo Elfving.

Budgeting and Priorities

Like any other crash and death countermeasure, renewing and extending pavement markings costs money. In budgeting and decision-making, much depends on how the purpose of reflectorized center lines and edge lines is viewed. If they are recognized as the prime frontline crash countermeasure they have proven to be, there is little doubt that funds will be allocated for their installation and maintenance. However, if the purpose of the lines is believed to be only for channelization and guidance, then the importance is diminished and other uses of limited funds might be made. The lobbyists for construction contractors have no shortage of alternative uses for funds. According to them, they would solve all safety issues with redesign and rebuilding of road infrastructure, an alternative far more expensive than that of pavement marking.

Construction and maintenance items dominate much of the discussion in budget preparation at highway departments. Road markings have no local, state or federal level partisans or lobbyists to compete with those of the construction contractors. Those responsible for installing and renewing the markings, and those interested in having them installed and renewed, must be their own advocates in budget preparations.

The supreme achievement of road construction contractors at the federal level in the United States was the establishment of the Highway Trust Fund in 1956. A tax of three US cents per gallon (now 18.4 cents per gallon) of gasoline sold was deposited into this repository. It was to fund construction mainly of the Interstate Highway System and the Federal Aid Highway System. The American Road and Transportation Builders Association (ARTBA) protested when money from the trust fund was proposed for road safety use. These road safety funds included money for pavement marking, spot improvements, obstacle removal and rail crossing provisions of the Highway Safety Act of 1973. While the overall Federal Aid Highway Act of 1973, of which the road safety act became a part, provided over US $10 billion for road construction, it seemed that construction contractors told their lobbyists to also get what money they could from funds set aside for safety. Some US $225 million allocated annually for other than pavement marking was available for road safety use.⁷

For each marking season throughout the rich world, contracts (or tenders) specifying roads to be marked, and standards and specifications to be met, are detailed in requested bids distributed to road-marking contractors. Many governments find it easier to contract out this work than to train and manage their own people and equipment in a task increasingly dominated by advanced technologies. Some larger marking contractors are noted for professionalism and for advancing marking technologies with ongoing research and development.

In this contracting scenario, the involvement by governments in executing any particular project can be reduced to that of a procurement agent. In many countries, the management of the procurement process and the contracts is complicated by the use of procurement departments with limited knowledge of pavement marking. Because of the usual requirement to accept the lowest bid for a particular project, there have been ongoing issues with the quality of the work. Some countries are reviewing the perceived need to accept a bid simply because it is the lowest, and are looking for ways to assure their public gets quality markings that last.

When governments do their own marking, they buy paint and beads by specification and usually in large quantities. With their own trained work forces and equipment, they are able to plan their own marking renewal campaigns without having to detail them in contracts and wait for the contracts awards process to be finished. This assures the timeliest possible response to renewal needs and it makes the highway departments responsible for the resulting quality of the lines.

The concepts of pavement marking related to crash reduction have to be brought to the attention of all involved in each of the processes of marking roads. From those responsible for budget allocations to those procuring pavement marking services, materials and equipment to the crews working in the field, all must understand that keeping pavement markings in good condition is very important work. The reason for pavement markings is not simply to provide guidance for car and truck drivers, but more importantly for reducing road traffic crashes, injuries and deaths.

7

Perspectives on Road Traffic Safety

Road traffic safety issues affect most people across the globe. The dimensions of road safety are immense, making it almost too big to grasp fully. The United States is a model of how large these dimensions are. Out of a population of 316 million, there were 212 million licensed American drivers in 2013. They had 269 million vehicles to drive, including 8.4 million motorcycles. Every year about four million new drivers are licensed. Every year somewhat fewer than four million die or don't renew their licenses. In America, there is more than one vehicle for every driver.[1]

The dramas played by these drivers are staged daily on 4,309,000 km (2,678,000 miles) of paved and 2,243,000 km (1,394,000 miles) of unpaved roads.[2] Of this amount, 103,000 km (64,000 miles) are limited access roads of the Interstate System or other expressways and toll roads; 647,000 km (402,000 miles) are arterial highway; and 1,297,000 km (806,000 miles) are collector highways.[3] These carried 86% of the traffic in 2013.[4] Local roads and streets comprise 4,602,000 km (2,860,000 miles), of which about half is unpaved.[5] If all of the American drivers lined up their cars or other vehicles on the paved roads, there would be one every 20 meters (22 yards).

Using 2013 as a typical year, there were about 1,591,000 traffic injury crashes and 30,057 crashes involving fatalities in America. In these, 22,383 vehicle occupants, 4,735 pedestrians, 4,668 motorcyclists, 743 bicyclists and 190 other/unknown died. A total of 2,313,000 were injured. Reducing these numbers is the primary purpose of traffic safety efforts. In addition, there were 4,066,000 crashes in which only property damage resulted, which could also benefit from reduction efforts. The core problem just in America is to influence the 212 million drivers to avoid more of the roughly 5.7 million annual crashes or to minimize the number who get hurt or killed.[6] Every other nation has its own dimensions with the same goal, with their particular scale and circumstances. The circumstances in Western Europe are similar to those in the United States.

The Elements of Traffic Safety

The earliest traffic safety efforts focused on getting irresponsible drivers off the road – those who would aggressively zoom their way through traffic speeding excessively. Only governments could establish reckless-driving laws and authorize speed limits and traffic controls. Ordinances about speed, driving in lanes and obeying traffic controls were generally left to be done by authorities closest to drivers at the provincial, state, district or local level. Intersections were equipped with signals or stop signs. Lanes were marked to guide traffic flow. Police arrested reckless drivers and those driving under the influence of alcohol or drugs. They also gave summonses to speeders and those who violated traffic rules like the right of way in intersections, lane usage, and passing only in designated passing zones.

Driver licensing was instituted so the driving privilege could be regulated for visual and other capabilities and for the license to be withdrawn for enforcement reasons. Subsequently, driving records were kept. The threat of cumulative penalties for speeding and other violations, including loss of license, were restraints on those unable to resist breaking the driving laws. At least that was the intent.

Also from early dates, vehicles were registered with license plates issued with identifying numbers. Stickers indicated if the plates and registration were current. Vehicle inspection was instituted to enforce vehicle safety standards. Lights, signals and brakes had to work. Conditions unsafe to the vehicle owner and the public at large were to be detected.

More recently, seatbelt use laws have been enacted. With enforcement of this type of law, government moved from not only trying to prevent crashes but also to increase the chances for survivability when a crash occurred. State and federal mandates, standards and funding for emergency medical services were also instituted.

Governments around the world promoted safe driving, safe walking and crossing of streets. Educational programs evolved, starting with teaching very young children about pedestrian and vehicle occupant safety. Films were made. Advocate and action groups appeared locally, regionally and nationally. Some corporate interest was aroused. Dialogue in America and Western Europe about road safety was ongoing from the 1920s onward. Deaths and injuries on the roads were not left without action to try to reduce them.

Most of these countermeasures were in place when deaths on American roads began to increase after 1961. Pushed by increases in car ownership and vehicle miles driven, road traffic fatalities rose by 50% over the following years to 1972.[7] As this occurred, federal, state and local governments sought answers as to how to prevent more deaths. Largely, they heard from advocates who urged more of the same solutions as in previous years, with improved national road safety standards and the addition of driver education for high school students and others. Ralph Nader and his devotees popularized information about unsafe automobiles while calling for federal regulation of automobile design. Also voiced was the idea that road deaths and injuries might have to increase as a price of modern life.

Advancements in Traffic Safety Thinking

The causes of road crashes have been discussed at academic institutions, in academic and engineering publications and in popular media. Bad weather, particularly with icy conditions or with snow descending, can wreak havoc on the roads. Cars and trucks crash and pedestrians fall. Emergency rooms can be overloaded. Drivers cannot do much when conditions are hazardous except to stay off the roads.

There is, however, general agreement on one basic reality. The cause of most crashes is due to drivers making mistakes. The reasons for the mistakes include fatigue, emotional upset, other distractions, or one too many beers or cocktails. The issue is how to prevent as many as possible of the potential mistakes from becoming actual mistakes that result in crashes, injuries and deaths.

Seeking means to stop and reverse the increases in road traffic fatalities in America, the US Highway Safety Act of 1973 changed focus to improving the safety of existing roads. It promulgated road safety engineering. This was a marked departure from the road user behavior modification approach embodied in the Highway Safety Act of 1966. At the time, the 1966 act reflected global thinking that all would be well if drivers obeyed the laws and did not drive while impaired.

With the new ideas promoted in the 1973 act, the roads got reflectorized center lines with passing zones and edge lines and intersections got new or improved signs and signals. Crosswalks were installed; road alignment and limited sight distance locations were treated, and rail-crossing hazards were upgraded. These actions are immediately effective to help drivers avoid crash-causing mistakes. Center lines and edge lines clearly show the direction, curves and elevation of roads, together known as "the alignment" of roads. Adding markings for passing zones further aids this alignment awareness signaling safe passing. The lines give positive guidance, being in continuous eye contact with drivers by day and especially at night. Their safety effectiveness has been tested and is well known, as discussed in Chapters 2 and 5. Installing full road markings on the United States rural roads of the federal aid system had a huge impact between 1973 and 1985. This led to fewer mistakes by drivers with the result of reduced crashes, injuries and deaths.

When drivers approach changes in alignment too fast, like in curves and particularly at night, if roads are center-lined and edge-lined, the radius and banking of the curve, and any change in elevation, will be reasonably visible. More drivers will slow down and negotiate the curve safely than would be the case if reflectorized lines were not there. When crashes start to happen, often by driving off the road, center lines and edge lines can help drivers better see a means of recovery for a possible safe ending. The same is true after an unexpected incursion by another car or truck, a cyclist, a pedestrian or an animal. Also, edge lines separate pedestrians from vehicle traffic, where there are no sidewalks, providing them with safer walking on the road edge.

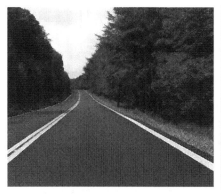 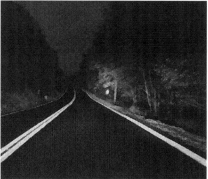

Figure 7.1[8]. *Rural road with center lines and edge lines shown in daylight.*   **Figure 7.2**[9]. *The same rural road at night.*

Research of the effectiveness of center lines and edge lines points to driving off the road to the right (in countries driving on the right) as a common first event in crash scenarios. The essential function of reflectorized longitudinal road markings is to prevent this from happening by aiding drivers to stay on the road and in the correct driving lane.

The United States and Western Europe experienced the success of road safety engineering. Improving the standards of existing roads showed very clearly that priorities of action is key to reducing road traffic crashes. Doing the things that produce results quickly only makes sense. Improving existing roads is paramount to accomplishing this. And so it is with Vision Zero and the safe system approach. Those contemplating and developing the concepts have a clear vision of the role of the road in road traffic safety.

The Vision Zero and the safe system concept expands on road safety engineering in that the road infrastructure is viewed as an integral part of the highway safety equation, with an aim to perfect it. Vision Zero aims to achieve a road system with no fatalities or serious injuries. Proponents would maximize the use of opposite-direction lane separation and intersection controls to prevent crashes. Extensive use of guardrails would minimize injuries resulting from cars leaving the roadway. Broad use of pavement marking would be universal. A strong social stigma against drinking and driving would be developed, with concurrent laws and regulations. Rigid licensing procedures, nearly 100% seatbelt use and helmet use, and a high measure of access to emergency medical service with the latest in mobile and hospital equipment, are additional features of achieving low death rates with this safe system approach.

Follow-on Actions to Road Safety Engineering

The American experience in reducing road traffic crashes, injuries and deaths did not end with road safety engineering. Following this success with improved roads, there was a targeted, long term and successful crash reduction effort discouraging impaired driving. Another effort targeted increased crash survival by promoting seatbelt use. These two campaigns, in addition to the road safety engineering efforts, are what is known to have worked in the United States and elsewhere in the rich world to reduce traffic fatalities.

Improving the safety of roads should always be a frontline step of any crash reduction campaign. Since many drivers are impaired by alcohol, fatigue, distraction or advancing age, helping them avoid crashes also means keeping other drivers, motorcyclists, bicyclists and pedestrians with whom they might collide, safe from harm. When all of the potential aids to help impaired drivers to avoid crashes have been achieved, the next step is then to reduce the number of impaired drivers on the roads.

To reduce impaired driving means getting drivers to modify their behavior and avoid impairment. The only tool governments have to do that is to influence drivers to obey traffic laws. Laws governing alcohol use while driving were in place in the USA early in the new motorized age, but were regularly disregarded. Enforcement has a limited effect as drunk drivers, lacking full reasoning, don't expect to make errors to draw attention from the police. Another kind of national effort was needed.

When Candace Lightner's teenage daughter was killed by a drunk driver in 1980, Ms. Lightner devoted the balance of her life to the campaign that created Mothers Against Drunk Driving (MADD) which impacted on the issue. The response she achieved led to the establishment of Ronald Reagan's Presidential Commission on Drunk Driving. Abiding by driving laws and enforcement thereof were emphasized. But mainly, the national campaign led American society to believe that driving after too much drinking was socially unacceptable. The idea of choosing a designated driver when needed was established. Something of the social stigma present in some Western European societies was implanted. Friends, hosts and hostesses could ask for the car keys of anyone seemingly unable to drive safely.

The results of the MADD campaign, aided by the Presidential Commission and the National Highway Traffic Safety Administration (NHTSA), have been measured by the number of deaths caused by alcohol-impaired driving. Such deaths have fallen by 11,000 (52%) from 1982 to 2013.[10] Pavement marking installations and the MADD campaign may have interacted since by 1985 road markings were in place throughout the US helping all drivers, but especially those impaired. The main thrust of the American campaign to discourage drinking and driving did not get started until 1982. Between then and 1985, about 3,000 fewer deaths caused by alcohol-impaired driving occurred.[11] Some of these lives saved could well have been attributed to the new road markings.

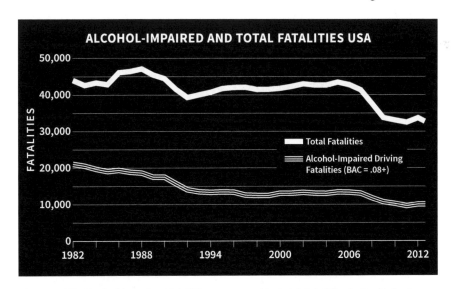

Figure 7.3[12]. *Alcohol-impaired fatalities compared to total fatalities in the United States 1982-2012.*

The seatbelt campaign was led by NHTSA marshaling the states to pass, promote and enforce laws requiring buckling up. These were met with a strange resistance at first. Seatbelts began appearing in American cars in the late 1950s and the three-point belt was ordained in 1974. By 1983, only 14% of drivers were using their seatbelts.[13] Drivers and passengers were not easily persuaded, but laws, and the work done to measure the effectiveness of seatbelts, were gradually accepted. The first state to require seatbelt fastening, New York, did so only in 1984.[14] In 2013, seatbelt use measured 87% in the USA, whereas in much of Western Europe, 95% or more used the restraints.[15,16] Failure to use a seatbelt is still the reason for many traffic deaths.

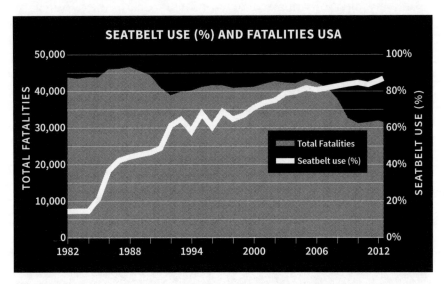

Figure 7.4[17]. *Total road traffic fatalities in the Unites States and percent of seatbelt use.*

The Highway Safety Establishment View

A mystifying remaining issue is why few contemporaries in the highway departments of the world, and fewer in the road traffic safety professions, seem to recognize the role of pavement marking as a primary crash countermeasure. It appears that a generation of road traffic safety practitioners has grown up in high-income countries without knowing how very important pavement markings are. Further, there seems to be a notable lack of awareness of the role road safety engineering played in reversing the road traffic fatality increases in the mid 1970s to the mid 1980s.

In high-income countries, the norms of road traffic safety were fixed from the early auto age. They were instinctive. It only made sense that driver and pedestrian behavior had to be improved by education, persuasion or penalty. These ideas developed in use and without very much oversight or testing. The traffic safety literature of the day was largely opinion. It is possible that the urgency of dealing with mounting road fatalities and injuries made action more important than analysis. The early public interest in pavement markings and their effect on traffic safety was never the subject of serious academic inquiry.

The instincts of those leading traffic safety and crash prevention efforts at the time carried forward programs based on these instincts. It was obvious that speed limits, traffic controls, prohibitions of reckless driving, limits on impaired driving, and later the use of seatbelts, were required. As early road safety organizations were established around newly motorized societies, the dogma from the 1920s was to preach safe driving, safe walking and enforcement of safety laws. Legislative action for traffic regulation was accordingly scripted. Enforcement in response to driver mistakes was rigorous and reached toward terrorizing miscreants in some nations. Drivers were mostly considered at fault in crashes. Various impairments of drivers were studied and alcohol was recognized at the forefront of these. Legally allowable blood alcohol content (BAC) levels were established and often reduced. Licensing requirements became stricter as the years advanced. Then car manufacturers were blamed for unsafe cars.

The academic literature on road safety was sparse. There was little questioning and less analysis and testing prior to the Federal Highway Administration (FHWA) research of fatalities by road system starting in 1967. Effectiveness research was rare. As the increase in road fatalities throughout the rich world manifested after 1960, rapidly growing traffic was blamed for increased fatalities despite declines in the death rate per distance traveled. There were laments that increases in fatalities and injuries would be the destiny of motorized societies. Such was highway safety before 1973.

With publicity absent in the media, other than speculations about when reductions in road deaths might appear, the continued attempts by the road-safety establishment to reverse increases in road deaths in high-income countries used mainly behavior modification approaches until the early 1970s. With little media attention, it is understandable how a momentous change in road safety policy and effectiveness happened without due notice and with a limited historical record. The classic tests of reflectorized center lines and edge lines described in Chapter 2 did not begin until 1952, some 40 plus years and two world wars after motorized transport began. Although the test results were initially ignored, eventually they would decisively change public policy regarding road traffic safety in high-income countries.

In the USA, the Highway Safety Act of 1966 added a new layer of bureaucracy to road safety. Newly established Governors Highway Safety Representatives in each state were mandated to review all policy and other actions to make sure they were compatible with newly established road safety standards. They in turn formed a national organization that focused on driver behavior interventions.

To the proponents of this kind of thinking, ideas that the physical roadway is an aspect of traffic safety and needing improvement and investment, were almost heresy. The Governors Highway Safety Representatives, and others involved with the traditional driver behavior modification programs, truly believed those programs would work if given time. Other powerful opposition to road safety engineering in America came from the road construction contractors bent on defending every dollar in the highway trust fund for grading, steelwork, cement, asphalt, gravel and their related services. They prophesized that only reconstruction of roads would bring reduced crashes and deaths.

When the new concepts of road safety engineering appeared in the draft Highway Safety Act of 1973, protests from the road safety establishment and the road builders vibrated around Washington. The Governor's Highway Safety Representatives, in hearings about the bill, openly preferred that the new, and large, sums allocated to road safety action programs be redirected to the states for their traditional programs. They claimed that they had reduced the death rate per million vehicle miles traveled although the total fatalities still increased.[18] Bill Harsha commented saying he thought reducing the total traffic deaths was the objective. Franklin Kreml, then President of the Motor Vehicle Manufacturers Association (MVMA), remarked to the committee that "we have not, as you know, gentlemen, achieved the success that was promised when the 1966 highway safety legislation was enacted."[19]

The administrative level of the Federal Highway Administration (FHWA), at the behest of the White House, asked in these hearings that there be no funding of road safety programs originated by the Committee on Public Works. Bill Harsha lost patience with them. He told them openly he thought they seemed not to be genuinely concerned with road safety.[20] He had spent much time studying the new ideas and was convinced of the crash and fatality reduction effectiveness of pavement markings. Most of the FHWA professionals, as opposed to the administrative level, agreed, supporting the development of the new road safety engineering projects and the funding allocated for them. The road construction lawyers and lobbyists pressured Harsha to back down. He did not.

Harsha, with the support of the senior members of the committee, effectively took control of road traffic safety policy in America. One of the senior members was James C. Wright, Jr., Democrat of Texas, who was to become Majority Leader and then Speaker of the House. Harsha understood that changes were needed and with the committee members caused them to happen. He rebuffed appeals by the Governor's Highway Safety Representatives and the objections of the White House of Richard Nixon. The bill, the Highway Safety Act of 1973, HR 2332, was co-sponsored by every member of the committee, making it fully bipartisan. The Senate passed its version of the bill by voice vote. When the bill became law as part of the Federal Aid Highway Act of 1973, little notice appeared in the press, nor did any noticeable professional analyses come forth.

No one in the group that Harsha and his staff gathered thought at the time that they were making road traffic safety history by emphasizing the role of roads in the road safety equation. It was not until ten years later that the results were evident in the reduction of fatalities on America's rural roads as described in Chapter 3. By then, Harsha had left Congress, Dick Peet had left the committee staff, Walter May and Richard Sullivan had retired and sadly, Lloyd Rivard had died. There were few staff or committee members remaining who were involved with the Highway Safety Act of 1973 to claim its success. Some papers appeared, but a meaningful conversation about the results of road safety engineering and pavement marking never got started.

By not later than the end of 1985, the rural and urban arterial and collector roads in high-income countries all had reflectorized center lines and edge lines installed and regularly maintained. All urban areas had lane lines, crosswalks and pedestrian islands. Some had bike lanes. The high population death rates declined somewhat, with reductions in crashes and deaths. The US rate fell from 26.1 in 1972 to 18.4 in 1985 with 9,000 fewer annual deaths on rural roads, where the road safety engineering and the pavement marking programs were focused.[21] Much more progress still lay ahead in the United States, Western Europe and in other high-income countries. A sound start was finally accomplished. It had taken a while.

In the story of the Federal Aid Highway Act of 1973, the importance of this large step forward in road traffic safety was eclipsed by an even larger step forward for funding mass transit expenditures. This new act was famous, or infamous, for allowing some of these expenditures to be paid from the Highway Trust Fund. This new transfer of funds instead became the subject of press conferences, speeches at various venues and hundreds of news articles. The liberal establishment had lobbied hard for this new funding for advancing or rebuilding the very expensive commuter railroads, the similarly expensive metro rail systems and bus and light rail routes. The immediate opportunity to develop public and academic interest in road safety engineering, and its potential as a road crash and death countermeasure, was lost in the perceived excitement about using the trust fund for mass transit expansion in cities and suburbs. Nobody in the United States' Congress or at the FHWA called press conferences or arranged presentations about the new road safety measures.

Lessons Encountered and Winning Public Support

The powerful story this book tells of the success of road safety engineering and pavement marking as key crash countermeasures apparently was substantially lost until now. Before that understanding faded, however, the practice of road safety engineering and adding pavement markings, spread throughout high-income countries. These concepts were quickly adopted in Western Europe. The marking of their roads was completed sooner than in the United States and those nations enjoyed the benefits sooner. As a result, hundreds of thousands of men, women and children were not killed or injured in crashes that did not happen.

Around the world, after the initial road safety engineering actions in the mid 1970s, there were opportunities for articles to be written about the successes. Publicity and articles about the resulting crash, injury and death reductions would have helped. A worldwide conversation about effective traffic safety action might have been started. A book about road safety engineering would have been helpful. Nothing much happened. Whether this failure of communication and documenting can be blamed is moot. It happened. Even in the formal American traffic manuals, there is no description of the key importance of road markings, especially of center lines and edge lines, as road traffic crash countermeasures.

It is very clear in a 1973 dialogue between Bill Harsha and Howard Pyle, President of the National Safety Council in the United States, and others, that public apathy regarding traffic safety in America was limiting progress. It was hard to get the attention of drivers to use seatbelts and to not drive while impaired. Franklin Kreml of the MVMA specified the lack of private sector support as a reason for the inadequate progress. He said support from industry, the media and the public was necessary to assure public acceptance of the road safety programs:[22]

"Public acceptance of these actions is not automatic. Resentment builds quickly when measures are applied without public understanding."

The Executive Director of the American Association of Motor Vehicle Administrators (AAMVA), Louis Spitz, took this a step further. In testimony for the 1973 act he said:[23]

"AAMVA is convinced that citizen participation is imperative if highway safety is to become a true national priority of the dimensions commensurate with the problems it causes."

He reported on the inauguration of a new road safety organization, STATES, Safety Through Action To Enlist Support. It was a federation of 29 national and state organizations with several million members organized to promote public support for the full implementation of the federal highway safety standards in each state.[24]

With some conjecture, there is a possible scenario by which public support in the United States for road safety programs was built. During the increase of American road traffic fatalities in the 1960's and early 1970s, over two-thirds of the yearly toll was on rural roads off the Interstate System. In 1973, it was clear that 1.3 million kilometers (800,000 miles) of mostly rural roads in the United States were not marked with center lines and edge lines. Further, there were several thousand intersections with no traffic controls. Drivers had some regulatory guidance as to which cars would go first, like priority given to the car on the right. Few in this 21st century will recall, or even imagine, the rudimentary conditions.

Beginning after the 1973 act, the new road safety programs brought evident change. Of the 122 million total American drivers in 1973, 80 million were age 30 and over and had been driving for at least 10 years.[25] Regular rural road users were mostly commuting to and from work or school or running personal errands. A proportion of them was cynical about government action or stayed in the margins of society. Many did not vote in elections. Their focus was on providing livelihoods for their families. Some held farm property; others lived in rural areas for the lower cost of living; yet others preferred the rural, small-town life made available to them by the new Interstate Road System or other new or expanded roads. Other rural road users were frequent passers-through from urban center to urban center or to sites of recreation. For many of these people, government appeals for safe driving were not a high personal priority. Those active in society saw increases in road fatalities nationally and locally with no evident progress or plan to reverse this trend. There was growing acceptance believing that nothing could be done because nothing meaningful was being done.

Mostly within five years, those drivers, having used the prior unmarked roads and driving through prior untreated intersections, saw newly installed reflectorized center lines and edge lines and newly erected signs and mounted signals. Their driving environment was transformed. These improvements were modestly publicized by highway departments. Local media paid more attention. Those who read newspapers, listened to the radio or watched TV news took interest. Even the cynics who did not read newspapers, or listened to the radio or watched TV news noticed the improvements. The conjecture is that the evident improvements, and the good results with road safety engineering in just a few years, got popular attention and was enough to motivate cooperation in further programs of limiting impaired driving, increasing the use of restraints and other actions.

In the developing world, with various levels of corruption, there is much more cynicism about government action. There is also more concern for day-to-day issues such as providing for personal and family livelihoods. For governments in these nations to embark on a major program to reduce road traffic tragedy is risky. Road safety engineering, however, deliver short-term results.

It is not conjecture that a meaningful road safety program will require public support for success. Achieving that support will not be easy. Where safety improvements are needed, road safety engineering can provide evidence of action to win public support. It will also deliver tangible short-term results to be publicized for building further support. Initial success will be important, and likely very significant, for building momentum for ongoing road safety programs.

8

The Story in Low- and Middle-Income Countries

Reducing road traffic tragedy in low- and middle-income countries remains an urgent issue. As set forth in the introduction, global road traffic fatalities in 2013 reached 1.25 million. Only about 125,000, or 10%, were in high-income countries, which had 46% of registered vehicles.[1] As previously noted, there has never before been traffic carnage of this magnitude. Only world wars surpass it in human cost.

At the peak of tragedy on the roads of 23 high-income OECD countries in 1972, there were about 170,000 fatalities and 4.3 million injuries.[2] Today, low- and middle-income countries are dealing with over six times as many fatalities and injuries annually. Also alarming in low- and middle-income countries is the buildup of disabled men and women. This annual toll is estimated at 5% of the number of injury crashes.[3] At a level of 25 injury crashes per fatality (the rate at the peak of fatalities in 1972 for high-income countries), about 1.4 million victims are permanently crippled in some way every year.[4] Over a 25-year generational period, this burden adds to 36 million incapacitated individuals. The costs compound annually.

A look at the raw dimensions of the issue is in the 15 low-and middle-income countries with the largest number of fatalities listed in Table 8.1. These countries have 65% of global annual fatalities and 60% of the population. They have an average death rate per 100,000 population of 22.5, ranging from 12.3 to 36.2. They have 45% of global registered vehicles and seven of them reported more motorcycles and mopeds than cars.

More raw dimensions are in Table 8.2 showing the 15 low- and middle-income countries (with populations over four million) who have the highest population death rates. They have 11.4% of global

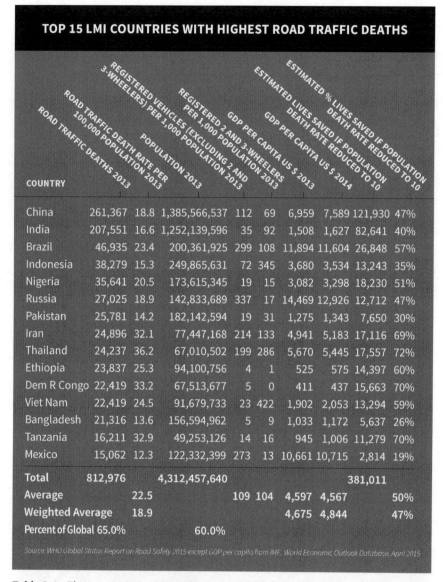

Table 8.1. The top 15 Low- and Middle-Income Countries with the highest road traffic deaths.

annual fatalities and 6% of the population. Of those reporting, five of the countries had larger registrations of two-wheeled than four-wheeled vehicles. They had 4.2% of total registered vehicles.

Tables 8.1 and 8.2 represent the cold facts of the road traffic safety situation in low- and middle income nations. The average

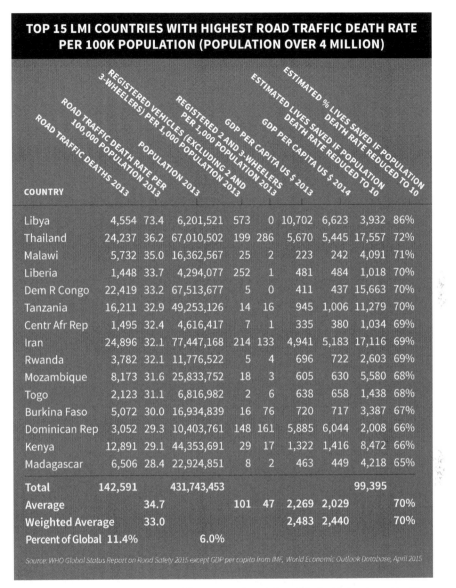

COUNTRY	ROAD TRAFFIC DEATHS 2013	ROAD TRAFFIC DEATH RATE PER 100,000 POPULATION 2013	REGISTERED VEHICLES (EXCLUDING 2 AND 3-WHEELERS) PER 1,000 POPULATION 2013	REGISTERED 2 AND 3-WHEELERS PER 1,000 POPULATION 2013	ESTIMATED % 3-WHEELERS	GDP PER CAPITA US $ 2013	GDP PER CAPITA US $ 2014	ESTIMATED LIVES SAVED IF POPULATION DEATH RATE REDUCED TO 10	ESTIMATED % LIVES SAVED IF POPULATION DEATH RATE REDUCED TO 10
Libya	4,554	73.4	6,201,521	573	0	10,702	6,623	3,932	86%
Thailand	24,237	36.2	67,010,502	199	286	5,670	5,445	17,557	72%
Malawi	5,732	35.0	16,362,567	25	2	223	242	4,091	71%
Liberia	1,448	33.7	4,294,077	252	1	481	484	1,018	70%
Dem R Congo	22,419	33.2	67,513,677	5	0	411	437	15,663	70%
Tanzania	16,211	32.9	49,253,126	14	16	945	1,006	11,279	70%
Centr Afr Rep	1,495	32.4	4,616,417	7	1	335	380	1,034	69%
Iran	24,896	32.1	77,447,168	214	133	4,941	5,183	17,116	69%
Rwanda	3,782	32.1	11,776,522	5	4	696	722	2,603	69%
Mozambique	8,173	31.6	25,833,752	18	3	605	630	5,580	68%
Togo	2,123	31.1	6,816,982	2	6	638	658	1,438	68%
Burkina Faso	5,072	30.0	16,934,839	16	76	720	717	3,387	67%
Dominican Rep	3,052	29.3	10,403,761	148	161	5,885	6,044	2,008	66%
Kenya	12,891	29.1	44,353,691	29	17	1,322	1,416	8,472	66%
Madagascar	6,506	28.4	22,924,851	8	2	463	449	4,218	65%
Total	142,591		431,743,453					99,395	
Average		34.7		101	47	2,269	2,029		70%
Weighted Average		33.0				2,483	2,440		70%
Percent of Global	11.4%		6.0%						

Source: WHO Global Status Report on Road Safety 2015 except GDP per capita from IMF, World Economic Outlook Database, April 2015

Table 8.2. *The top 15 Low- and Middle-Income Countries with the highest road traffic death rate per 100,000 population (Population over 4 Million).*

2014 GDP per capita for all of the countries in these two tables is below US $5,000. The columns representing the potential lives saved if the population fatality rates are reduced to 10 in these countries, the approximate current rate of the United States, is roughly what is needed in order to cut global fatalities

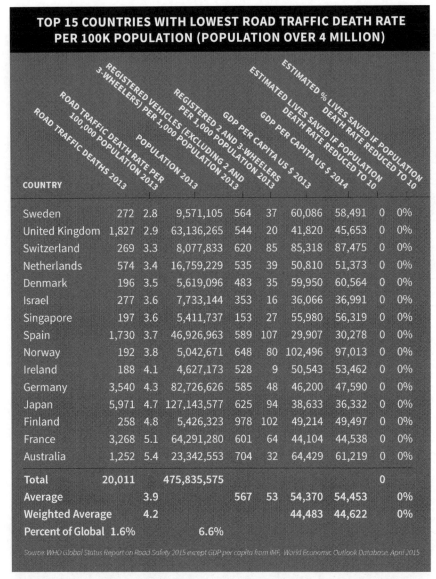

TOP 15 COUNTRIES WITH LOWEST ROAD TRAFFIC DEATH RATE PER 100K POPULATION (POPULATION OVER 4 MILLION)

COUNTRY	ROAD TRAFFIC DEATHS 2013	ROAD TRAFFIC DEATH RATE PER 100,000 POPULATION 2013	REGISTERED VEHICLES (3-WHEELERS) PER 1,000 POPULATION 2013	REGISTERED 2 AND 3-WHEELERS PER 1,000 POPULATION 2013	GDP PER CAPITA US $ 2013	GDP PER CAPITA US $ 2014	ESTIMATED LIVES SAVED IF DEATH RATE REDUCED TO 10	ESTIMATED % LIVES SAVED IF POPULATION DEATH RATE REDUCED TO 10
Sweden	272	2.8	9,571,105	564	37	60,086	58,491	0	0%
United Kingdom	1,827	2.9	63,136,265	544	20	41,820	45,653	0	0%
Switzerland	269	3.3	8,077,833	620	85	85,318	87,475	0	0%
Netherlands	574	3.4	16,759,229	535	39	50,810	51,373	0	0%
Denmark	196	3.5	5,619,096	483	35	59,950	60,564	0	0%
Israel	277	3.6	7,733,144	353	16	36,066	36,991	0	0%
Singapore	197	3.6	5,411,737	153	27	55,980	56,319	0	0%
Spain	1,730	3.7	46,926,963	589	107	29,907	30,278	0	0%
Norway	192	3.8	5,042,671	648	80	102,496	97,013	0	0%
Ireland	188	4.1	4,627,173	528	9	50,543	53,462	0	0%
Germany	3,540	4.3	82,726,626	585	48	46,200	47,590	0	0%
Japan	5,971	4.7	127,143,577	625	94	38,633	36,332	0	0%
Finland	258	4.8	5,426,323	978	102	49,214	49,497	0	0%
France	3,268	5.1	64,291,280	601	64	44,104	44,538	0	0%
Australia	1,252	5.4	23,342,553	704	32	64,429	61,219	0	0%
Total	20,011		475,835,575					0	
Average		3.9		567	53	54,370	54,453		0%
Weighted Average		4.2				44,483	44,622		0%
Percent of Global	1.6%		6.6%						

Source: WHO Global Status Report on Road Safety 2015 except GDP per capita from IMF, World Economic Outlook Database, April 2015

Table 8.3. The top 15 Countries with the lowest road traffic death rate per 100,000 population (Population over 4 Million).

in half per the 2030 agenda for Sustainable Development Goals.

For comparison, the 15 high-income nations (with populations over four million) with the lowest population fatality rates have an average rate of 3.9. These countries have 6.6% of the world population, but 17.6% of the world's registered vehicles. They only have

1.6% of global, annual fatalities. Their average 2014 per capita GDP is about US $44,600.

Low- and middle-income countries differ from each other as much as they do from high-income countries. Some have traffic divisions and highway departments led by professionals with degrees from top rated colleges and universities. Many are dedicated to their jobs and to advancing national and societal interests, but others are, or will become, corrupt. In some countries, traffic is wild, with irresponsible drivers ignoring traffic laws, signs and signals. Traffic laws, vehicle registration or licensing requirements are sometimes incomplete. Traffic enforcement may be by well-trained and well-motivated men and women or it may be incomplete or corrupt. In some countries, needed road improvements are not accomplished for lack of political will or from lack of, or misappropriation of, funds.

As our narrative has shown, high-income nations went through the same trauma of high road traffic fatality rates now experienced in low- and middle-income countries. The United States had a death rate per 100,000 population of 26.1 in 1972; Austria had 40.2; France, 35.2; Canada, 28.0; Germany, 27.0; Italy, 22.1; Japan, 19.3; Sweden, 14.7 and the United Kingdom 14.5.[5] The high-income nations inaugurated successful countermeasures. The path was neither easy nor smooth. Along the way, even as fatalities kept increasing, most theoreticians and advocates of traffic safety argued for continued efforts to change driver behavior and enforcement as the only solutions. Those in leadership roles pleaded for more time to allow traditional actions to change driver behavior. Then, in the United States, research of traffic fatalities by road system from the Federal Highway Administration (FHWA) appeared. As a result, some began to realize that the enormous efforts to change human behavior since the 1950s had missed something. It became clear that there might be issues with the roads. A small but highly influential group in the United States then turned policy emphasis to the roads and road safety engineering as described in Chapter 3.

The United Nations' Efforts

The United Nations visibly took action on the matter of the global increases in road traffic crashes, injuries and deaths in 2004. The torch was handed to the World Health Organization (WHO), a UN agency, to lead this effort through its Department for Management of Noncommunicable Diseases, Disability, Violence and Injury Prevention. There seemed to be no other suitable UN agency to assume leadership even though road traffic safety, under Injury Prevention, is not a good fit. To help in the road traffic safety endeavor, the WHO set up the United Nations Road Safety Collaboration (UNRSC). It is described as "an informal consultative mechanism whose members are committed to road safety efforts."[6] In 2009 a second and smaller ad hoc group was formed, The Friends of the Decade of Action for Road Safety 2011-2020. It is described as "an informal group of governments and international agencies committed to making the Decade a success."[7] Even though there is no specific roster, this group has been instrumental in shaping the political agenda that lead to the declaration of the Decade of Action in May 2011 and the development of its Global Plan. This group seems to meet once or twice a year with the purpose of advising and supporting the WHO. It is difficult to determine how the WHO or the UNRSC or the Friends of the Decade are accountable for anything they do or for reaching any proclaimed objectives or targets.

The first major work, *World Report on Road Traffic Injury Prevention*, was produced jointly by the WHO and the World Bank in 2004.[8] This effort, 244 pages of academic prose, seemed intent on accommodating every known reference. There was particular emphasis of the perceived relationship between public health and road safety. The report was prepared in an unusual way. There were 17 editors, but no acknowledged authors. Rather, there were technical committees of no less than five members who were in some way responsible for each chapter. There were peer reviewers and other advisors lending input. Who was accountable and for what in the report is not clear. The report seems more like an aggregation of different facts, ideas and anecdotes, sometimes contradictory, without contributing much of meaningful analyses or conclusions. Indeed, critical facts were missed.

The purpose of this 2004 report, as it stated, "is to present a comprehensive overview of what is known about the magnitude, risk factors and impact of road traffic injuries, and about ways to prevent and lessen the impact of road crashes."[9] The report also stated: "It is hoped that the launch of this report will mark the beginning of a long process of improving road safety. If it is to be effective, the report should stimulate discussion at local, national and international levels, and the recommendations should serve to bring about greatly increased actions on road traffic injury prevention around the world."[10]

Whatever the intent, the report caused very little real action. Road traffic crashes and deaths in developing nations did not abate.

By 2009 the need for a reappraisal was evident. A new *Global Status Report on Road Safety, Time for Action*, was prepared by the WHO.[11] This time the report was 54 pages of discussion followed by a single-page country profile compiled from self-administered questionnaires completed by each of 178 countries, plus a statistical index of 61 pages. Bloomberg Philanthropies provided the funding. This report delivered information from each country, but it still missed the essentials of the experience of the rich world in combating road traffic crashes and deaths focusing on improving the safety aspects of existing roads.

An inaugural Global Ministerial Conference on Road Safety was held in Moscow also in 2009. The Decade of Action for Road Safety 2011-2020 program was proclaimed and Bloomberg Philanthropies provided US $125 million in funding for the first five years of the program aimed at 10 selected countries. A Global Plan for the Decade of Action for Road Safety 2011-2020 was prepared by the WHO together with the UNRSC.[12] During this decade, the program was to save five million lives on the world's roads. This implied global fatalities would be reduced by 2.5 million to approximately 900,000 annually.[13]

The Global Plan for the Decade of Action recommends 34 activities and 48 sub-activities, presenting an assortment of road safety options but without offering any priorities for proposed actions. These activities are divided into five "pillars": (1) Road Safety Management; (2) Safer Roads and Mobility; (3) Safer Vehicles; (4) Safer Road Users; (5) Post-Crash Response. It calls for nations to establish a single lead agency to take control of all road safety activities, to be followed by the development of a national strategy with long-term commitments of investment.

As it is, the effect of the Global Plan on low- and middle-income countries is to complicate their tasks. The plan prescribes overly complex options without recommending priorities. The following quotes represent this. The full text is available on the WHO website and can be downloaded in six languages.[14]

> "Experience suggests that an adequately funded lead agency and a national plan or strategy with measureable targets are crucial components of a sustainable response to road safety."

> "Effective interventions include incorporating road safety features into land-use, urban planning and transport planning; designing safer roads and requiring independent road safety audits for new construction projects; improving the safety features of vehicles; promoting public transport; effective speed management by police and through the use of traffic-calming measures; setting and enforcing internationally harmonized laws requiring the use of seat-belts, helmets and child restraints; setting and enforcing blood alcohol concentration limits for drivers; and improving post-crash care for victims of road crashes. Public awareness campaigns also play an important role in supporting the enforcement of legislative measures, by increasing awareness of risks and of the penalties associated with breaking the law."

> "[The Global Plan] is intended as a guiding document for countries, and at the same time for facilitating coordinated and concerted action towards the achievement of the goal and objectives of the Decade of Action for Road Safety 2011–2020. It provides a context that explains the background and reasons behind the declaration of a Decade by the United Nations General Assembly. This Global Plan serves as a tool to support the development of national and local plans of action, while simultaneously providing a framework to allow coordinated activities at regional and global levels. It is directed at a broad audience including national and local governments, civil society and private companies willing to harmonize their activities to-

wards reaching the common objective while remaining generic and flexible to country needs."

Very little of this dialogue is tangibly associated with reducing crashes, injuries and deaths. Totally absent is any reference to, or analysis of, how the rich world succeeded in reducing their road traffic fatalities. Also missing is any discussion or advice regarding the role of the existing road infrastructure and how it can be made safer with short-term results. It seems that somehow, the safety condition of the existing road infrastructure is not actively viewed as an integral part of the whole road safety issue.

As the Global Plan includes high-income countries in its scope, it makes the plan and its recommendations mostly impractical for low- and middle-income countries. The route to incremental gains in road safety by high-income nations is vastly different from initial and ongoing gains needed in low- and middle-income countries. Since the goal was to save 500,000 lives annually from roadway death, and only about 125,000 total lives are lost in high-income countries, it seems the plan must have been intended mostly for low- and middle-income countries. Why then was the plan not focused on helping these countries specifically with appropriate advice and countermeasures? Although the intent of the Global Plan is good, it lacks focus and priorities of action to be of real assistance.

In 2013, the WHO published the 318 page *Global Status Report on Road Safety 2013, Supporting a Decade of Action*.[15] The information builds on the 2009 Global Status Report and its format and is based on 2010 data. It was to serve as a baseline to monitor and evaluate the Decade of Action program. Bloomberg Philanthropies again provided financial support for the report. A total of 1.24 million annual fatalities were enumerated with no overall reductions. Eighty-eight countries were reported to have decreased fatalities, but another 87 countries had increases.[16]

The same language and suggestions from prior publications appear. Road traffic safety is still promoted as a public health issue. Without being specific, statements like "strong evidence base on what interventions work" are used. The related focus on pushing for increased legislation on the five key risk factors – speed, drink-driving, motorcycle helmets, seatbelts and child restraints – that the WHO seems to have settled on being the most important, continues. That 35 countries adopted new laws on one or more of these five key risk factors is touted as concrete progress.[17] Appropriate legislation, and enforcement thereof, is important, but it is not enough to seriously make any substantial progress. What is still missing is actionable advice on how to meaningfully reduce road traffic crashes, injuries and fatalities.

In the fourth year of the Decade program, late in 2014, the WHO was able to report that some nations have established a lead agency for road safety and new or improved traffic legislation. Some had improved enforcement, some required helmets for motorcycle and moped riding, some required the buckling of seatbelts and the use of child restraints in vehicles. Others were conducting road assessments. And some were doing mass media campaigns and educating journalists.[18] But how many lives were saved and injuries avoided?

To raise the visibility of road safety as a worldwide issue, and hopefully to garner more meaningful road safety action, the UN Secretary General, Ban Ki-moon, announced the appointment of Jean Todt as his Special Envoy for Road Safety in April of 2015.[19] Mr. Todt is the President of FIA, Fédération Internationale de l'Automobile, a "global organisation that aims to safeguard the rights and promote the interests of motorists and motor sport all across the world."[20] Mr. Todt is also a trustee of the FIA Foundation for the Automobile and Society. This is a separate organization that "supports an international programme of activities promoting road safety, the environment and sustainable mobility, as well as funding motor sport safety research."[21] The main role of the Special Envoy will be to "help mobilize sustained political commitment at the global level towards making road safety a priority worldwide."[22]

In September of 2015, the UN adopted Sustainable Development Goals for 2030. For the first time, goals for road traffic safety were included. Specifically:[23]

> Under the category Good Health and Well Being: By 2020, halve the number of global deaths and injuries from road

traffic accidents.

Under the category Sustainable Cities and Communities: By 2030, provide access to safe, affordable, accessible and sustainable transport systems for all, improving road safety, notably by expanding public transport, with special attention to the needs of those in vulnerable situations, women, children, persons with disabilities and older persons.

The UN/WHO appears to anticipate that including road traffic safety in the agenda for the 2030 Sustainable Development Goals will get it more global exposure and potentially open up additional access to funding. The goal to cut the number of global road traffic deaths and injuries in half by 2020 is very aggressive. This goal is unattainable unless the UN/WHO dramatically changes their approach to the problem. The act of setting a goal, especially without having a concrete plan to accomplish it, is not by itself progress. More funding for existing and mostly behavior modification countermeasures will not produce the needed results.

In October of 2015, a follow-up report came from the WHO, *Global Status Report on Road Safety 2015*.[24] In 340 pages, similar in language and format to the 2013 report, it aims to summarize the current road safety situation and highlight the progress made over the past three years. Globally, a total of 1.25 million road traffic fatalities were reported, a seeming plateauing compared to the 2013 and 2009 WHO reports, with 79 countries seeing decreased fatalities, but another 68 countries seeing increases. Unfortunately for populations in low- and middle-income countries, the main progress claimed is that "In the last 3 years 17 countries, representing 409 million people, have amended their laws on one or more key risk factors for road traffic injuries to bring them into line with best practice."[25] The WHO also produced a highly condensed 16-page summary version of the report.[26]

In November 2015, the *Second Global High-Level Conference on Road Safety* was held in Brasilia, hosted by the government of Brazil and co-sponsored by the WHO. As stated before the conference, "Brazil would like to have a robust outcome document approved as a result of the Conference – the Brasilia Declaration – through a sound intergovernmental negotiation process involving consultation with other stakeholders."[27]

The reality was the Brasilia Declaration was drafted, in arduous UN language, already in early 2015 and opened worldwide for comment. Your authors addressed this clause in the draft:[28]

> "Noting that the overwhelming majority of road traffic deaths are avoidable, that at the mid-point of the Decade of Action insufficient progress has been made and that it is time to strengthen road safety policies and measures, recognizing that it is futile to only blame the victims of road traffic crashes and that there is a shared responsibility to move towards a world free from road traffic fatalities"

In the June draft of the document, this critical clause had been removed and was replaced with the following in the final document:[29]

> "Noting that the overwhelming majority of road traffic deaths and injuries are predictable and preventable and that at the mid-point of the Decade of Action much remains to be done, despite some progress and improvements in many countries, including in developing countries"

It appears that the WHO was very wary of any criticism of the Global Plan and their lack of progress. The conference planners seem to have established an agenda that would as much as possible sustain and applaud the work of the WHO and the Decade of Action thus far. The American vernacular for this is "whitewashing." No real report of the outcome of the conference has come forth from the WHO or the Brazilian organizers. The only official result from the conference has been the adoption of the Brasilia Declaration document that was prepared beforehand and is still written in arduous UN language.

The FIA Foundation published on their website what looks like a report on the conference but with a focus on their activities. The FIA report tells of "a powerful speech by the FIA Foundation's ambassador, road safety advocate and mother of a road traffic victim, Zoleka Mandela. Mandela told government ministers that there could be no more excuses for inaction. "No more empty commitments. No more delay. We are approaching five years into the Decade of Action for Road Safety. Road deaths are actually rising in nearly 70 countries. Where is the action? Where is the urgency?"[30]

The UN/WHO Failings

At this writing (early 2016), five years after the start of the Decade program, most of the nations concerned should have long been reporting reductions in crashes, injuries and deaths. High-income nations 40 years earlier paid dearly to learn what to do. After, or while, putting laws, ordinances, and enforcement in place, the task is to bring existing roads up to the highest possible safety standards without reconstruction. Much can be done quickly. Reflectorized center lines with passing zones and edge lines can be installed on all paved arterial and collector roads. Intersections can be newly signed and signaled or upgraded, as can rail grade crossings. Once these safety improvements are made, they are immediately effective at keeping some driver mistakes from becoming crashes and at separating pedestrians from vehicle traffic. The success in the rich world was based on this shift from a focus on changing road user behavior to improving safety standards of the existing road network.

There seems to have been a huge misunderstanding by the WHO of which road traffic crash countermeasures actually produced the results in high-income nations. The sharp declines in road traffic deaths from 1973 to 1985 on the roads of high-income nations did not result from a robust adoption of behaviorist policies or from safety regulations of auto designs. Rather, reduced fatalities resulted primarily from road safety engineering actions that improved existing but safety deficient roads. It was not until the road safety improvements were in place that campaigns for discouraging drinking before driving, encouraging buckling of seatbelts and other road user behavior based countermeasures became effective. These took 30 years to show meaningful results, more than a generation.

There also may be a cultural barrier inherent in the makeup of the WHO. Since its founding in 1948, it has taken a public health view on global issues. In 1962, there was a WHO paper by L.G. Norton, and further writings by Dr. William Haddon Jr., which put forth a philosophy proclaiming road safety to be a public health issue, that road traffic injury is equivalent to disease and suggesting a concept of epidemiology to solve it.[31] It was enticing to think that interventions typical of public health might reduce road traffic tragedy.

This concept of epidemiology was aimed at driver and pedestrian behavior. The public health category actions of passing laws and regulations, processing and enforcing them and urging behavior change seemed to fit. In countering disease, laws and proper behavior work. But in dealing with road safety, there is much more to it than that. By 1970, new research in the United States by the FHWA showed dramatically different crash results on different road systems. It was a powerful realization that the conditions of the roads were critical variables in the road safety equation and whether or not crashes could be prevented. It was also a realization that the locus of road safety happens on roads of varying types: rural, urban, arterial or collector; in daylight, dawn, dusk or night; with traffic light, moderate or heavy; crawling or at typical urban or rural speeds. There is little in public health or medicine that pretends to deal with the prevention of crashes on real roads. In the end, the idea of some kind of epidemiology did not seem to fit with reality.

As crashes occur on roads of various types with traffic of various types, speeds and volumes, the first priority remedy is to improve the roads to help drivers avoid crashes. Enforcement of traffic laws, proper court procedures, advanced driver training, strict licensing standards, and detailed vehicle inspections are not subjects in medical or nursing schools or in university public health curricula. How to calm traffic, design lanes for powered two-wheelers, separate pedestrians, regulate intersections and organize traffic crash data are not taught there either. The role of treating road traffic crash injuries, like any other injury, is medical, but the prevention of such crashes is not. No nation successful in minimizing traffic deaths and injuries has ever given that responsibility to a public health agency. It is certainly questionable as to why such is being advised on a global scale.

Also, the WHO seems to only acknowledge in theory the concept of a "safe system" approach to road traffic safety. As stated, for example, in the concluding chapter of the 2004 report, the WHO promotes a safe-system approach to road safety: "Any road traffic system is highly complex and hazardous to human health. Elements of the system include motor vehicles, roads and road users, and their physical, social and economic environments. Making a road traffic system less hazardous requires a "systems approach" – understanding the system as a whole and the interactions between its elements, and identifying where there is potential for intervention." Further in the same chapter the WHO states: "Many high-income countries have shown sharp reductions in crashes and casualty numbers over the past couple of decades. This has been achieved by adopting a systems approach to road safety that emphasizes environment, vehicle and road user interventions, rather than solely focusing on direct approaches aimed at changing the behavior of road users."[32]

In reality, the WHO has mostly ignored the impact roads have in the road traffic safety equation and hence mostly omits promoting proven countermeasures dealing with the road network. The WHO has positioned itself as the global leader and expert in road safety and as such advises the global community on what it considers best practices and proven countermeasures. The advice they promote is mostly limited to that of a public health lens. This focus is on five key risk factors: speed, drink-driving, motorcycle helmets, seatbelts and child restraints. These are all behavior modification countermeasures with potential results mainly in the long-term. Also, the long-term, nation-building, capital-intensive activities promoted in the Global Plan lack priorities and are out of reach for most low- and middle-income nations in the short-term. Instead, these nations need a simplified series of priorities of actions that will produce immediate results. These can be implemented in nations where there is strong political will and leadership at the national level to improve road traffic safety.

Recommended Priorities for
Low- and Middle-Income Countries

High-income countries never produced anything as complex as the WHO Global Plan, but they learned that plans do not gain traction without road safety engineering first generating quick and significant results. In the best example of this, the United States and Western Europe spent large amounts on campaigns to get people to obey the laws, to establish road safety standards about everything, and to promote traffic safety across society. Deaths on America's roads, and on those in Western Europe, still continued to increase. Public discouragement about the lack of results in reducing road traffic crashes and deaths led to comments such as risking your life on the roads might have to be the price to pay for modern life.

Road safety engineering finally appeared on the American scene in 1973. As described here in Chapters 3 and 7, it was encouraged from, and enacted at, the very highest levels of the American government. That swept aside less viable options suggested by other advisors and promoted by their advocates. There was at last some funding to focus traffic safety on the roads. Analysis found two-thirds of the fatal crashes in the United States were on rural two-lane roads. There were no center lines and edge lines on most of them. As the retroreflective lines were installed on 1.3 million kilometers (800,000 miles) over twelve years, there was at the end a 35% decrease in deaths on these rural roads while deaths on urban roads increased by 17%.[33] Further action started programs of spot improvements. This provided quick but long-term fixes to untreated or difficult intersections, dangerous road alignments, threatening roadside obstacles and inadequate sight distances.

The early experience of the United States, Western Europe, Japan and the well-to-do nations of the British Commonwealth indicates the Global Plan needs to be amended, or a separate plan altogether needs to be developed, to provide for priorities of action. The plan also needs to be simple. Here are eight priorities that will produce real results. Start with priorities One and Two and work on them in parallel. Preferably, also work on priorities Three and Four in parallel. In most circumstances, then follow the sequence as laid out below, but again considering working on more than one of the actions at the same time, depending on local circumstances. For priorities Five to Eight to make any real impact, priorities One and Two, and preferable Three and Four as well, need to be in place as a base to build on:

PRIORITY 1: Establish traffic laws and enforcement means thereof and related authorizations and enforcements for rules and ordinances.

Firm laws must prohibit reckless and aggressive driving and a mandate given to enforcement with severe penalties. Similarly, limits to define driving impaired by alcohol and drugs need to be set and enforcement organized and trained. Policy concerning speed limits, intersection controls, center line passing zones, lane lines, stop signs and bars, lanes for two-wheeled vehicles, and pedestrian crossings should establish the basis for ordinances and guides to enforcement. Police training, compensation and management should be aimed to mitigate corruption and raise effectiveness. Helmet, seatbelt use and child restraint laws should be established as well as meaningful annual vehicle inspections. Laws and enforcement for on-the-spot vehicle road-worthiness inspection (working brakes, lights etc.) and vehicle overcrowding must also be established. Driver licensing and vehicle registration should be set up or updated with a uniform records system. All laws, policies and other action must be publicized continually and shared with other parties included in road safety programs.

PRIORITY 2: Maximize the safety of existing roads with road safety engineering.

While legal and enforcement actions are being developed or implemented, begin road safety engineering actions to raise the safety standards of the existing road system. Set up crash data gathering as needed and conduct surveys to establish plans of action and budgets. Install reflectorized center lines with passing zones and edge lines on all paved arterial and collector roads. Test and install bicycle lanes; pedestrian lanes, footpaths and road crossings; and motorcycle lanes where possible. Test urban lane markings for traffic calming. Select intersections and rail highway grade crossings to be treated and install signs and signals as needed. Publicize the reason for all projects and improvements and especially the results.

PRIORITY 3: Establish a capable road traffic safety data system.

Set up a central organization for the uniform collection of traffic safety data. Develop collection means in every police station, emergency room and first responder base enabling tabulation of crash locations, time of day and types of crashes; persons killed and injured; alcohol and drug involvement; and seatbelt or helmet use. Develop audit capability and procedures to enhance accuracy. Provide incentives for staff and others to comply and to do so consistently.

PRIORITY 4: Establish a first responder network.

Build a network of on-road medical, fire and police rescue services to provide crash victims with emergency first-aid and for transporting them to medical treatment facilities. Establish a plan for funding, communications and legal framework for cooperation among first responders and healthcare providers.

PRIORITY 5: Establish campaigns to end driving under the influence of various drugs and alcohol.

Publicize the legal BAC percent limits and enforcement intentions and penalties. Engage print and broadcast media and social media. Develop campaigns with organizations promoting designated drivers, social responsibility and other actions discouraging impaired driving. Enlist aid of celebrities. Set up web sites and provide educational materials. Promote the use of designated drivers and the idea that drinking and driving is socially unacceptable behavior.

PRIORITY 6: Establish campaigns to promote the wearing of helmets by all two-wheeled vehicle drivers and their passengers.

Continuously publicize the importance of using helmets, that the helmets must functionally provide adequate protection, and enforcement intentions and penalties. Organize supply and distribution as necessary.

PRIORITY 7: Establish campaigns for the use of seatbelts and child restraints.

Continuously publicize the benefits of using seatbelts and child restraints, enforcement intentions and penalties. Build cooperation with organizations that will assist. Require all cars to have three-point seatbelts.

PRIORITY 8: Establish campaigns to continually promote safety in driving, walking, and two-wheeled riding.

Develop staff to conduct safety promotion for good driving, safe motorcycling, safe bicycling and safe walking. Use education, print and broadcast media and social media for a continuous stream of information. Continually measure and evaluate effectiveness and results.

Much of the WHO Global Plan is entangled in issues far beyond that of road traffic safety. Infrastructure development, including expanded transportation, land use planning, capacity planning and establishing healthcare facilities, will eventually have to be taken into consideration when they can be financed and paid for, but short-term improvements in road safety can be accomplished less expensively with road safety engineering. As even mentioned in the Global Plan, an incremental approach to develop a national road safety strategy will be needed in some countries. Implementing road safety engineering improvements is an effective and proven first step in such an approach. With the magnitude of global road traffic fatalities, real action for something to happen immediately is needed. There are ways to accomplish this without first having to create a full-fledged national plan or to entirely trying to rebuild low- and middle-income countries.

The immediate need to reduce road traffic injuries and fatalities in low- and middle-income countries makes most of the Global Plan moot in the short-term. Until those nations with population death rates of 20 or more get them down to 10 or less, primary consideration should be given to the reduction of road traffic crashes and deaths by first addressing the safety standards of existing roads. Then join that with campaigns to reduce the number of impaired drivers on the roads, to increase the number of buckled seatbelts and worn helmets and for reducing speeds. Until significant progress has first been realized with these countermeasures, not much attention should be focused on new structures, new thoroughfares, new transport means or new healthcare facilities.

Likewise, focusing work on improving safety standards of vehicles in low- and middle-income countries, except to establish realistic safety inspections of existing vehicles, is not going to produce any meaningful reductions in road traffic crashes, injuries or fatalities in the short-term.

The eight priorities outlined above are the recipe for what a country looking to reduce road traffic deaths and injuries needs to do and in what order. However, to make the Global Plan, or any plan for that matter, successful, adequate funding and political will at all levels – global, national and local – are necessary.

The Role of the Rich World

Those nations with per capita GDP of over US $40,000 that render aid to nations with a GDP of less than US $4,000, need to consider the road traffic tragedy these countries suffer very seriously. No industrialized nation would tolerate the levels of cost and loss most of these countries endure. High-income countries might consider traffic deaths in low- and middle-income nations to be solely their local problem. High-income countries, however, export cars, trucks, busses, motorcycles, mopeds and all kinds of other products and services to these countries. They are important growth markets.

There are two main economic issues related to road traffic crashes, injuries and fatalities in developing countries. The first is that the resulting economic cost endured by these nations make up a significant percentage of their annual funds available for discretionary spending and productive investing. This then affects the ability of a country to grow economically and its future ability to purchase factory equipment, computers and related electronics, hospital equipment, construction cranes and materials and other exports from high-income countries.

Of 125 low- and middle-income countries, 42, ranging in population from Jamaica (2.8 million) to India (1.25 billion), provided their estimated costs of road traffic crashes as a percent of GDP. Using 2014 GDP numbers from IMF, of the 42 reporting countries, there were six low-income nations that averaged US $1,859 per crash; 16 lower middle-income nations averaged US $12,470 per crash; and 20 upper middle-income nations averaged US $42,255 per crash. Extrapolating the average costs from these income groups to the full number of countries in each income group shows that low- and lower- middle-income nations lose 2.75% of their GDP to road crashes. As described in the introduction, this annual toll is a large portion diverted from investment where only shallow amounts of GDP may be available annually to make life better in these countries. Reducing the impact of road traffic crashes as much as possible as quickly as possible is very much is order to stop this diversion of scarce resources. In upper- middle-income nations, the loss due to road traffic crashes is 2.3% of GDP.[34]

The second main economic issue related to road traffic crashes in low- and low- to middle-income countries was first raised at the International Road Federation meeting in Brazil in 1984. It is speculative, but the dialog on this point has continued. In these nations, educated and skilled men and women are scarce. Elite, professional and other families able to do so, send their young people to Western universities that welcome them, often with scholarships. Many then go on to lives and careers in high-income countries where life is more comfortable and surely safer than at home.

Those who are required to return to their home country, or who feel the calling of their homeland, are especially valuable. They work in business, government, healthcare, education, social work and in universities. They are more likely to be driving or motorcycling and in doing so, they are more exposed to being involved in road traffic crashes. For a nation to not have the appropriate countermeasures in play may lead to wasting especially valuable citizens who get killed or become disabled.

The UN and the WHO need to feel the pressure from high-income nations to push for real progress in reducing road traffic crashes in low- and middle-income countries. But few high-income countries have shown any real interest in this global issue. It is, however, high-income nations that have the experience of knowing what to do and in what order. They can supply equipment and expertise. They can also chip in with financial aid for road safety projects as part of their current foreign aid programs.

New goals also have to be set for low- and middle-income countries. Influence and pressure from high-income nations is needed to refocus the UN, the WHO, the World Bank and others on actions that will produce short-term results. Twelve years have passed since 2004. Roads are not becoming much safer and casualties are still mounting. Some insisting needs to be done, as does some assisting. High-income countries need to act wherever there is evident political will at the national and local levels to fully deal with the aggregate road safety issue with practical and proven means.

While we speak of road traffic tragedy as a cost measured in percent of a nation's GDP, and in using other clinical terms, there is the human dimension. As related in the introduction, road traffic safety statistics are not abstract numbers. The figures represent uncountable grief at untimely death, disrupted families and social units, suffered and treated injuries, and a build-up of men, women and children with permanent disabilities. All this pain, anguish, frustration, and trauma are in addition to financial loss. This human dimension of suffering once was a reason by itself for action by those with the means to take action.

Setting priorities of action that will produce meaningful results in reducing road traffic tragedy, and securing funding for those actions, are the ultimate objectives for low- and middle-income nations. Joined to that is achieving the political will at all levels to push through these required actions.

Conclusion

The decisions that led to the road safety engineering actions in America in 1973, to be followed in Western Europe and elsewhere in the rich world, were landmark. Very quietly, but emphatically, the focus of road crash, injury and fatality reduction shifted from broad attempts to influence drivers to behave perfectly to raising the safety standards of existing roads to help keep their mistakes from becoming crashes. Roads were center-lined and edge-lined where needed. Intersections of various types got signs, signals, stop bars and crosswalks. Rural and urban road alignments, roadside environments, and sight distances were improved.

Over hardly more than a decade, almost all of the arterial and collector roads in the United States and Western Europe were upgraded with predictable results, based on tests of crash, injury and fatality reduction on both sides of the Atlantic. Road safety engineering proved to be a dramatically effective crash countermeasure tool. As reflectorized center lines and edge lines were renewed, and roads were otherwise maintained, the safety benefits continued. It was a momentous shift in road safety policy throughout high-income countries. The Vision Zero aim for a perfected road system later expanded this to the "safe system" approach to road traffic safety.

The goal of road safety engineering is to prevent road traffic crashes. This is essential. If a crash does not happen, then no one has to survive it. If the number of crashes is not reduced, traffic tragedy will still increase despite potential better odds of crash survivability. As crashes happen on roads, resulting from driver mistakes, the condition of the road is critical from a road traffic safety perspective. Unlike countermeasure actions regarding road user behavior and vehicle safety standards, all road users benefit from safer roads immediately when improvements are made.

Getting existing roads up to the best possible standard without rebuilding them is the purpose of road safety engineering. These measures provide initial and immediate results and require no conscious behavior modification by road users. Once completed, and as long as the improvements are maintained, crash reductions continue to accrue. As a potential crash countermeasure in low- and middle-income countries, this passive characteristic of road safety engineering should be especially attractive. Then, leveraging on that base of crash reductions, campaigns to discourage drinking and driving, to encourage buckling seatbelts and for other actions that all take more time, can more readily follow successfully. No program aimed at reducing road traffic crashes and fatalities has been successful without first implementing road safety engineering.

Road safety engineering to improve existing roads was adopted in the rich world and was mostly completed by 1985. There was little academic involvement. Few analyzed, commented on or enlarged upon the classic tests or the accomplished results. There were limited publications, but journalists generally did not follow these events. The publicity of the time was about vehicle crashworthiness and smashing up cars, Ralph Nader and William Haddon Jr. being the apostles. Much was claimed by the car safety regulators in terms of fatality reduction, but the reality was that vehicle crashworthiness did not prevent a single crash. Crashes were mainly prevented by implementing road safety improvements that kept driver mistakes from becoming serious or tragic events.

One purpose of this book is to emphasize the fact that road safety engineering with reflectorized road markings is the most effective, and likely the most affordable, crash countermeasure on two-lane roads. The authors of the comprehensive COST 331 study completed in 1999 by the European Commission found that road marking is "one of the most effective (i.e. with one of the highest cost-benefit ratios) low cost engineering measures available for improving road safety."[1] Similarly, summarizing a meta-analysis study by the Institute of Transport Economics in Oslo, Norway shows that when the combination of center lines and edge lines are added to roads, total crashes are reduced by 24%, a significant drop.[2]

For the most part, the road safety community of the era opposed road improvement measures. They felt deeply that behavior change was the only solution. They also did not want to lose potential funding to a new "upstart" idea. Highway contractors and road builders also opposed the use of public funds for road safety engineering, wanting the money spent on their projects, building new roads and bridges. Bill Harsha and his congressional supporters, however, prevailed in pushing through funding of substantial road safety improvements to existing roads in the United States. Similar opposition to road safety engineering is still prevalent. To the detriment of populations in the developing world, this opposition favors a continued focus mainly on behavior modification countermeasures, on building new roads, on improving vehicle safety and on providing alternate means of transportation. No nation has been successful in reducing road traffic tragedy with such a limited approach.

Getting to Road Traffic Fatality Reductions

Another purpose of this book concerns road traffic tragedy in the developing world. The fundamental need in the developing world is to reduce road traffic crashes, injuries and fatalities on existing roads as soon as possible. This means starting road safety engineering, most importantly by putting down reflectorized center lines and edge lines and installing and maintaining signs and signals. Further to that is the need for accurate data. The development of data collection and analysis capabilities is an essential part of road traffic safety to track progress or analyze the lack thereof. Implicit is the need for capable staff, equipment and systems. Most developing countries will need assistance.

The World Health Organization's *Global Plan for the Decade of Action for Road Safety 2011-2020* seems to exclude road safety engineering activities and misses the need for priorities of action.[3] In the conclusions and recommendations of the *Global Status Report on Road Safety 2015*, there is evidence of the intent to marginalize the role of existing roads in road traffic safety planning.[4] It is clear that the advice is focusing on attempting to modify road user behavior and on regulating vehicle safety standards. This is an inadequate approach for the developing world. It fails to include the critical countermeasure tools of road safety engineering. The importance of the safety condition of the existing road infrastructure should not be filtered out of primary consideration. The WHO also fails to recognize the need for public involvement and support.

The truth is that current road traffic tragedy is occurring on current road infrastructure, with a current vehicle mix, and in nations with a current level of healthcare access. Within these current parameters, countermeasures to reduce road traffic crashes and deaths must provide the largest and most immediate results at a cost these nations can at least contemplate affording. The WHO Global Plan prescribes overly complex and long-term options without recommending priorities of action. This type of long-term planning can happen in parallel, but the current road traffic crisis requires prioritized, proven, realistic and relevant countermeasures for short-term results. The priorities recommended herein set forth an order of action. It is reasonable to say that unless these priorities are enacted in the developing world, little progress can be expected.

Planning for road safety engineering needs to be accomplished with each nation separately that can demonstrate the requisite political will and leadership to support a road safety program. Governments, political entities and other involved organizations need to recognize that public involvement and support for the program is essential. Undertaking road safety engineering actions produces the needed short-term results on which to gain public notice and interest. Because equipment and training is integral to both road safety engineering and the data support, external foreign aid funding will move things along and indeed get programs started. Until basic safety improvements are made to existing roads, and until nations have trustworthy data, any progress in road crash reduction will be slow, if it even appears. The time has come for the rich world to chip in. Road traffic fatalities and injuries are impeding developing world economic growth.

A new entity responsible for global road safety, and with fully accountable leadership and competent staff that can solicit foreign aid funding from donor nations, needs to be established.

Such an organization might be part of the WHO or the UN or perhaps the World Bank or another global organization. It could be staffed by professionals from participating governments and from other sectors experienced in traffic safety or data. It would require funding sufficient to add to the capabilities of developing nations to undertake the priorities recommended herein. The size and complexity of projects, and how many nations to be helped at the same time, will determine the staff needed and how fast progress can be made.

Of the questions that might linger, the matter of urgency is paramount. Despite claiming urgency in many conferences and publications, nothing in the UN/WHO activities indicate urgency in action. With its fundamental misconception of what produced decreasing road traffic fatalities in the rich world, the UN/WHO got on the wrong track. Had the UN/WHO discovered the fact that road safety engineering had been the first priority of the successful phase of crash and fatality reduction in high-income nations, it would have made a huge difference in action and results in the developing world. Indeed, the goal of cutting fatalities in half might by now have been surpassed.

It is plausible that much of the incomplete and erroneous thinking by the UN/WHO, and for that matter also by much of the global road safety community, links back to labeling road traffic safety a public health issue. Road traffic safety, as a multi-dimensional issue, includes aspects of public health, but it is a road traffic safety issue, not a public health issue. In insisting that it is a public health issue, it has been reduced to one only dealing with and promoting solutions and countermeasures with which the public health community feels comfortable. Hence, the stated goal to reduce road traffic crashes, injuries and fatalities has been severely hampered by ignoring the road environment and any available countermeasures relating thereto. Making a measurable change in driver behavior takes years. Making a measurable change with improved vehicle safety standards and crashworthiness also takes years. Building new roads and bridges likewise takes years. Road safety engineering, however, is effective immediately and records results in weeks.

It is now time for the UN/WHO and the global road safety community to get on the right track. It is the experience of the rich world that building drink-driving or restraint use programs on the base crash reductions achieved first by road safety engineering is key for making these programs succeed. Road safety engineering also achieves the initial and visible results needed to gain the support of the public that is vital for success. If road safety engineering demonstration programs in developing world conditions are deemed necessary for funding of the proposed programs and actions herein, arrangements for this should be made expeditiously. Not only does road safety engineering produce short-term, but lasting, results, it also provides that much needed hope for the public that the tragedy now playing out on the roads can indeed be reversed. For the developing world, any results, but especially short-term results, are long overdue.

Authors' Note

Our focus with this book is on proposing what can be done now in low- and middle-income countries with proven, simple and prioritized actions implementable under existing conditions to reduce the road traffic tragedies occurring there. Longer term planning, taking into account a wider array of programs, ought to occur in parallel. However, the immediate need to reduce current road traffic crashes, injuries and fatalities is the issue at hand. The time spent by the UN and the WHO in proposing highly complex and structured planning articulated in the Decade of Action Global Plan has very likely led to large numbers of crashes, injuries and fatalities that might have been prevented had a more pragmatic approach been taken. Getting the simple and practical priorities going in developing nations should be the global priority. We have described the scientific basis for them in this book. The follow-on goal is to then really get down to work on implementing actions in countries with the political will to make a difference. Now is the time to move this decade-old discussion forward, towards real action.

Vehicle Safety Standards and Technology Advancements

We have purposely not expanded on, or touted, vehicle safety standards or new vehicle technology advancements in this book even though exciting things are happening in these areas. We certainly respect the importance of vehicle safety standards and that they should not be relaxed in vehicles sold in the developing world compared to those sold in rich countries. The regrettable reality, though, is that the value from improving vehicle safety standards or adding new vehicle safety technologies for conditions in low- and middle-income countries as means to reduce road traffic tragedies in the short-term is negligible.

The current (and unacceptable) numbers of crashes occur with vehicles already on the roads interacting with large numbers of two-wheeled and pedestrian road users. Improved vehicle safety, by the time standards are legislated and the vehicle fleet is renewed, is more than a decade away. Discussing improved vehicle safety standards and new vehicle safety technologies perhaps makes good copy in the rich world, but offers only marginal short-term, real-life improvements for the developing world. Work to improve vehicle safety standards in these nations is in order, but it should not consume much time or resources in the near term.

Academic Theories and Potential Countermeasures

We have also purposely not debated all conceivable countermeasures or academic theories of potential road safety actions. These might have an eventual place in improving road traffic safety in low- and middle-income countries, but the advancement and implementation of these will have to start in rich nations. Developing nations have a current and urgent need for initial and immediate progress.

Global Road Traffic Fatality Data

In our recommendations for assisting nations with a political will to take action, the two critical steps are initiating road safety engineering and establishing reliable and uniform data gathering and analysis capabilities. Distributions of road traffic fatalities by rural, urban, and limited access highway roads in night and daytime conditions focused attention in America on countermeasures related to the roads. Good data is necessary to guide progress in developing nations.

For lack of other sources of road traffic fatality information for low- and middle-income countries, we have used data from the different published WHO global status reports. The fatality rates in these reports are those based on the public health measure of population rather than on distance travelled. Data for distance travelled is not available for most countries.

The WHO has shown awareness of the need for data. Estimating algorithms for road traffic fatalities have been used by the WHO to try to reach comparable totals by nation. However, for the Global

Status Report on Road Safety 2015, the estimation methodology changed so that the 2015 estimates are not directly comparable to previous estimates published in prior status reports on road safety. There are also substantial differences between the WHO estimates and government reports in some cases. India is one example where the WHO estimated fatalities are 70,000, or 51%, higher than the fatalities reported by the government. If the data provided by the Indian government were to be proven accurate, the total global road traffic fatalities would be reduced by six percent. Globally, the WHO estimated fatalities are 94% higher than the fatalities reported by individual governments. In tracking progress, caution is needed to make sure compatible data with compatible estimating methods is used.

Acknowledgements

No intellectual product of this nature or magnitude is ever produced without profound assistance. During the course of researching and writing this book, many individuals and organizations all over the world lent their input and helped clarify issues and details. We are especially indebted to Robert Haru Fisher of Fisher Publications in New York. Bob was our editor, advisor and critic throughout the journey. Thank you, Bob, and thanks to everyone else. You know who you are.

If not for the continued support and patience of our wonderful ladies, Amie Brockway-Henson and Janis Elfving, this book would not have happened. This was their contribution to the future reduction of road traffic deaths and injuries. We love you and are deeply indebted to you.

Since this book is really just the beginning of an endeavor to reduce global road traffic tragedies, we would greatly appreciate any input, critiques and ongoing comments and help with spreading the word. Reach us at info@RoadSafetyRealities.com. You can find additional information at www.RoadSafetyRealities.com.

Gerry Balcar and Bo Elfving
Margaretville, New York
May 18, 2016

Notes

Introduction

1. World Health Organization. *Global Status Report on Road Safety,* 2015
2. ibid
3. ibid
4. IRTAD (International Road Traffic and Accident Database). Data extracted on 18 Feb 2015.
5. World Health Organization. *Global Status Report on Road Safety,* 2015 and International Monetary Fund, World Economic Outlook Database, April 2015. Downloaded August 15, 2015
6. ibid
7. World Health Organization. *Global Status Report on Road Safety,* 2015
8. IRTAD (International Road Traffic and Accident Database). Data extracted on 18 Feb 2015
9. World Health Organization. *Global Status Report on Road Safety,* 2015
10. Figure I.1. IRTAD (International Road Traffic and Accident Database). Data extracted on 18 Feb 2015
11. World Health Organization. *World Report on Road Traffic Injury Prevention,* 2004
12. World Health Organization. *Global Plan for the Decade of Action for Road Safety 2011-2020*

Chapter 1

1. Popular Mechanics, December, 1930. *First Speed Law in America*
2. Federal Highway Administration (FHWA). State Motor Vehicle Registrations 1900 – 1995. Table MV-200. April 1997
3. Historical Statistics of the United States, 1789-1945, U.S. Department of Commerce, Bureau of the Census, Series K 174-175 page 220, Washington, D. C., 1949
4. National Highway Traffic Safety Administration (NHTSA). Traffic Safety Facts – 2013 Data. July 2015
5. Federal Highway Administration (FHWA). Highway Statistics 2013, Table HM-12M
6. Federal Highway Administration (FHWA) and National Highway Traffic Safety Administration (NHTSA) historical data. Motor vehicle traffic fatalities & fatality rate: 1899 - 2003
7. Wikipedia. *https://en.wikipedia.org/wiki/Road_surface_marking*
8. Federal Highway Administration (FHWA). State Motor Vehicle Registrations 1900 – 1995. Table MV-200. April 1997
9. Historical Statistics of the United States, 1789-1945, U.S. Department of Commerce, Bureau of the Census, Series K 174-175 page 220, Washington, D. C., 1949
10. Federal Highway Administration (FHWA) and National Highway Traffic Safety Administration (NHTSA) historical data. Motor vehicle traffic fatalities & fatality rate: 1899 - 2003
11. Wikipedia. *https://en.wikipedia.org/wiki/Road_surface_marking*
12. ibid
13. Figure 1.1. "M-15 centerline 1917" by Unknown - Higher quality copy of photo courtesy of the Michigan Department of Transportation. Original publication in Kulsea, Bill (1980) Making Michigan Move: A History of Michigan Highways and the Michigan Department of Transportation, Lansing, MI: Michigan Department of Transportation, p. 10. Licensed under Public Domain via Commons - https://commons.wikimedia.org/wiki/File:M-15_centerline_1917.jpg#/media/File:M-15_centerline_1917.jpg
14. Figure 1.2. Rogers, Frank F. (1922) Biennial Report of the State Highway Commissioner for the Fiscal Years ending June 30, 1921, and June 30, 1922 (9th ed.), Lansing, MI: Fort Wayne Printing, p.6, plate I. Federal Highway Administration (1977) *America's Highways, 1776–1976: A History of the Federal-Aid Program,* Washington, DC: US Government Printing Office, p. 127 OCLC:

3280344. Licensed under Public Domain via Commons - https://commons.wikimedia.org
15. Wikipedia. *https://en.wikipedia.org/wiki/June_McCarroll*
16. Figure 1.3. *The Visual Link of Prevention*. Movie produced and copyrighted by Potters Industries, Inc. Written and directed by Gerald Balcar, 1982
17. Wikipedia. *https://en.wikipedia.org/wiki/June_McCarroll*
18. Figure 1.4. A German Autobahn in the 1930's. Source: Wikipedia. Public Domain via Commons. *https://commons.wikimedia.org/wiki/File:German_Autobahn_1936_1939.jpg*
19. The Institute of Transportation Engineers. *http://library.ite.org/pub/e1beddcd-2354-d714-5125-f6d6080ed36e*

Chapter 2

1. The German tests were conducted in German. English language summaries of the tests are from *The Advisor for Accident Prevention* published by the German Association of Liability and Accident Insurance Companies, Cologne 1961
2. Traffic Quarterly. April, 1955
3. Traffic Safety. September, 1957
4. The Hy-Lighter. Vol 1, No 5, Michigan State Highway Department, 1958
5. Traffic Accident Experience Before and After Pavement Edge Line Painting. State of Illinois Department of Public Works and Buildings, Division of Highways, Bureau of Traffic (Springfield: 1959)
6. Highway Research Board Bulletin 266, 1960
7. Highway Research Board Bulletin 308, 1962

Chapter 3

1. Federal Highway Administration (FHWA) and National Highway Traffic Safety Administration (NHTSA) historical data. Motor vehicle traffic fatalities & fatality rate: 1899 - 2003
2. ibid
3. Figure 3.1. Federal Highway Administration (FHWA) and National Highway Traffic Safety Administration (NHTSA) historical data. Motor vehicle traffic fatalities & fatality rate: 1899 - 2003
4. Insurance Institute of Highway Safety. Selected bibliography of William Haddon Jr., M.D., IIHS President 1969-1985
5. Figure 3.2. Haddon, William, Jr. Prepared for a presentation at the American Medical Association Conference on Prevention of Disabling Injuries, Miami, Florida, May 20, 1983
6. United States Public Law 89-564, Sept. 9, 1966, *Highway Safety Act of 1966*. http://www.gpo.gov/fdsys/pkg/STATUTE-80/pdf/STATUTE-80-Pg731.pdf
7. Federal Highway Administration (FHWA) and National Highway Traffic Safety Administration (NHTSA) historical data. Motor vehicle traffic fatalities & fatality rate: 1899 - 2003
8. Highway Safety Act of 1966. Hearings before the Committee on Public Works, House of Representatives, Eighty-ninth Congress, Second Session on H.R. 13290 and Related Bills. March 22, 23, 24, May 3, 4 and 5, 1966
9. United States Public Law 89-563, Sept. 9, 1966, Traffic and Motor Vehicle Safety Act of 1966. https://www.govinfo.gov/content/pkg/STATUTE-80/pdf/STATUTE-80-Pg718.pdf)
10. ibid
11. State of the Union Messages of the Presidents: 1790-1966 (New York: Chelsea House Publishers, 1967)
12. IRTAD (International Road Traffic and Accident Database). Data extracted on 18 Feb, 2015
13. United States Public Law 93-87, Aug. 13, 1973, Title II, Highway Safety Act of 1973. http://www.gpo.gov/fdsys/pkg/STATUTE-87/pdf/STATUTE-87-Pg250.pdf
14. Figure 3.3. Pocket Congressional Directory January 1973, Government Printing Office, Ninety-Third Congress, p. 113. http://babel.hathitrust.org/cgi/pt?view=image;size=100;id=m-dp.39015073070487;page=root;seq=125;num=113
15. Figure 3.4. Copyright Potters Industries, Inc. 1973 Highway Legislation (Highway Safety). Hearings before the Subcommittee on Transportation of the Committee on Public Works, House of Representatives, Ninety-third Congress, First Session on H.R. 2332 to Authorize Appropriations for Certain Highway Safety Projects, and for other Purposes. March 1, 6 and 7, 1973

16. Figure 3.5. Copyright Potters Industries, LLC. The Potters Brothers: An American Story 2014
17. Table 3.1. 1973 Highway Legislation (Highway Safety). Hearings before the Subcommittee on Transportation of the Committee on Public Works, House of Representatives, Ninety-third Congress, First Session on H.R. 2332 to Authorize Appropriations for Certain Highway Safety Projects, and for other Purposes. March 1, 6 and 7, 1973
18. Figure 3.6. Copyright Potters Industries, Inc. 1973 Highway Legislation (Highway Safety). Hearings before the Subcommittee on Transportation of the Committee on Public Works, House of Representatives, Ninety-third Congress, First Session on H.R. 2332 to Authorize Appropriations for Certain Highway Safety Projects, and for other Purposes. March 1, 6 and 7, 1973
19. Figure 3.7. Copyright Potters Industries, Inc. 1973 Highway Legislation (Highway Safety). Hearings before the Subcommittee on Transportation of the Committee on Public Works, House of Representatives, Ninety-third Congress, First Session on H.R. 2332 to Authorize Appropriations for Certain Highway Safety Projects, and for other Purposes. March 1, 6 and 7, 1973
20. Figure 3.8. Copyright Potters Industries, Inc. 1973 Highway Legislation (Highway Safety). Hearings before the Subcommittee on Transportation of the Committee on Public Works, House of Representatives, Ninety-third Congress, First Session on H.R. 2332 to Authorize Appropriations for Certain Highway Safety Projects, and for other Purposes. March 1, 6 and 7, 1973
21. 1973 Highway Legislation (Highway Safety). Hearings before the Subcommittee on Transportation of the Committee on Public Works, House of Representatives, Ninety-third Congress, First Session on H.R. 2332 to Authorize Appropriations for Certain Highway Safety Projects, and for other Purposes. March 1, 6 and 7, 1973
22. Figure 3.9. Copyright Potters Industries, Inc. 1981. Illustrations by Anthony Di Lorenzo
23. Figure 3.10. Copyright Potters Industries, Inc. 1981. Illustrations by Anthony Di Lorenzo
24. Federal Highway Administration (FHWA). Highway Statistics 1973-1985, Table VM-1
25. Federal Highway Administration (FHWA). Persons Fatally Injured in Motor Vehicle Crashes, 1967-1995. April 1997
26. ibid
27. Federal Highway Administration (FHWA). Highway Statistics 1973-1985, Tables VM-2 and VM-3
28. Table 3.2. Federal Highway Administration (FHWA). Persons Fatally Injured in Motor Vehicle Crashes 1967-1995. April 1997. Table FI-210
29. ibid
30. National Highway Traffic Safety Administration (NHTSA). Traffic Safety Facts
31. ibid
32. IRTAD (International Road Traffic and Accident Database). Data extracted on 18 Feb, 2015
33. National Highway Traffic Safety Administration (NHTSA). Traffic Safety Facts
34. ibid
35. World Health Organization. *Global Status Report on Road Safety,* 2015

Chapter 4

1. IRTAD (International Road Traffic and Accident Database). Data extracted on 18 Feb, 2015
2. European Commission, Directorate General Transport. Luxembourg: Office for Official Publications of the European Communities, 1999, ISBN 92-828-6506-1. *COST 331 Requirements for Horizontal Road Marking. Final Report of the Action.*
3. European Transport Safety Council (ETSC) Fact Sheet. *France: New Legislation to Tackle Alcohol as Main Cause of Road Deaths.* March, 2009. http://archive.etsc.eu/documents/Fact_sheet_Drink%20Driving%20France.pdf
4. ibid
5. Gizmag. *France's bold drink driving legislation – every car to carry a breathalyzer.* February 24, 2012. http://www.gizmag.com/france-breathalyzer-legislation/21541/
6. IARD.org (International Alliance for Responsible Drinking). http://www.iard.org/Policy/Policy-Resources/Policy-Tables-by-Country/Blood-Alcohol-Concentration-BAC-Limits
7. DinkDriving.org. http://www.drinkdriving.org/drink_driving_statistics_uk.php#convictionstatistics
8. IRTAD 2014 Annual Report © OECD/ITF 2014
9. Bussgeldkatalog 2015. https://www.bussgeldkatalog.org/alkohol-drogen/
10. HowToGermany.com. *DUI – Not a Good Thing* by Peter Horvath. http://www.howtogermany.

com/pages/expat2.html
11. Wikipedia - *Bob Campaign.* https://en.wikipedia.org/wiki/Bob_campaign
12. Wikipedia – *Seat Belt Legislation.* https://en.wikipedia.org/wiki/Seat_belt_legislation
13. World Health Organization Global Health Observatory Data Repository. http://apps.who.int/gho/data/view.main.51416
14. National Highway Traffic Safety Administration (NHTSA). Traffic Safety Facts 2009, Table 78
15. European Road Safety Observatory (ERSO). Traffic Safety Basic Facts 2011.
16. Wikipedia – *Drunk Driving Law by Country.* https://en.wikipedia.org/wiki/Drunk_driving_law_by_country#Europe
17. IRTAD (International Road Traffic and Accident Database). Data extracted on 18 Feb, 2015
18. eHow – *DUI Penalties in Australia.* http://www.ehow.com/list_6373966_dui-laws-australia.html
19. eHow – *DUI Penalties in Canada.* http://www.ehow.com/list_6114545_dui-penalties-canada.html
20. IRTAD (International Road Traffic and Accident Database). Data extracted on 18 Feb, 2015 and IARD.org (International Alliance for Responsible Drinking). http://www.iard.org/Policy/Policy-Resources/Policy-Tables-by-Country/Blood-Alcohol-Concentration-BAC-Limits

Chapter 5

1. Merrill J. Allen, Ph.D. *Vision and Highway Safety.* Chilton Book Company, Philadelphia, 1970
2. ibid
3. ibid
4. ibid
5. Figure 5.2. *The Visual Link of Prevention.* Movie produced and copyrighted by Potters Industries, Inc. Written and directed by Gerald Balcar, 1982
6. Figure 5.3. *The Visual Link of Prevention.* Movie produced and copyrighted by Potters Industries, Inc. Written and directed by Gerald Balcar, 1982
7. Figure 5.4. *The Visual Link of Prevention.* Movie produced and copyrighted by Potters Industries, Inc. Written and directed by Gerald Balcar, 1982
8. Figure 5.5. *The Visual Link of Prevention.* Movie produced and copyrighted by Potters Industries, Inc. Written and directed by Gerald Balcar, 1982
9. Figure 5.6. *The Visual Link of Prevention.* Movie produced and copyrighted by Potters Industries, Inc. Written and directed by Gerald Balcar, 1982
10. Figure 5.7. *The Visual Link of Prevention.* Movie produced and copyrighted by Potters Industries, Inc. Written and directed by Gerald Balcar, 1982
11. Figure 5.8. *The Visual Link of Prevention.* Movie produced and copyrighted by Potters Industries, Inc. Written and directed by Gerald Balcar, 1982
12. Figure 5.9. *The Visual Link of Prevention.* Movie produced and copyrighted by Potters Industries, Inc. Written and directed by Gerald Balcar, 1982
13. Nedas, N., Balcar, G., Macy, P. *Road Markings as an Alcohol Countermeasure for Highway Safety: Field Study of Standard and Wide Edgelines.* Abridgement published in Transportation Research Record 847, Transportation Research Board, National Research Council, Washington, DC, 1982
14. ibid
15. Figure 5.10. Nedas, N., Balcar, G., Macy, P. *Road Markings as an Alcohol Countermeasure for Highway Safety: Field Study of Standard and Wide Edgelines.* Abridgement published in Transportation Research Record 847, Transportation Research Board, National Research Council, Washington, DC, 1982
16. Figure 5.11. *The Visual Link of Prevention.* Movie produced and copyrighted by Potters Industries, Inc. Written and directed by Gerald Balcar, 1982
17. Figure 5.12. *The Visual Link of Prevention.* Movie produced and copyrighted by Potters Industries, Inc. Written and directed by Gerald Balcar, 1982
19. Figure 5.13. *The Visual Link of Prevention.* Movie produced and copyrighted by Potters Industries, Inc. Written and directed by Gerald Balcar, 1982
19. Nedas, N., Balcar, G., Macy, P. *Road Markings as an Alcohol Countermeasure for Highway Safety: Field Study of Standard and Wide Edgelines.* Abridgement published in Transportation Research Record 847, Transportation Research Board, National Research Council, Washington, DC, 1982
20. Figure 5.14. Nedas, N., Balcar, G., Macy, P. *Road Markings as an Alcohol Countermeasure for*

Highway Safety: Field Study of Standard and Wide Edgelines. Abridgement published in Transportation Research Record 847, Transportation Research Board, National Research Council, Washington, DC, 1982
21. Figure 5.15. Nedas, N., Balcar, G., Macy, P. *Road Markings as an Alcohol Countermeasure for Highway Safety: Field Study of Standard and Wide Edgelines.* Abridgement published in Transportation Research Record 847, Transportation Research Board, National Research Council, Washington, DC, 1982
22. Figure 5.16. Nedas, N., Balcar, G., Macy, P. *Road Markings as an Alcohol Countermeasure for Highway Safety: Field Study of Standard and Wide Edgelines.* Abridgement published in Transportation Research Record 847, Transportation Research Board, National Research Council, Washington, DC, 1982
23. Nedas, N., Balcar, G., Macy, P. *Road Markings as an Alcohol Countermeasure for Highway Safety: Field Study of Standard and Wide Edgelines.* Abridgement published in Transportation Research Record 847, Transportation Research Board, National Research Council, Washington, DC, 1982
24. European Commission, Directorate General Transport. Luxembourg: Office for Official Publications of the European Communities, 1999, ISBN 92-828-6506-1. *COST 331 Requirements for Horizontal Road Marking. Final Report of the Action.*
25. Timothy J. Gates and H. Gene Hawkins, Texas Transportation Institute, The Texas A&M University System, College Station, Texas. Research Report 0024-1 *The Use of Wider Longitudinal Pavement Markings,* 2002
26. ibid
27. ibid
28. ibid
29. ibid
30. ibid
31. ibid
32. Paul Carlson and Jason Wagner, Texas Transportation Institute, The Texas A&M University System, College Station, Texas. *An Evaluation of the Effectiveness of Wider Edge Line Pavement Markings,* 2012
33. ibid
34. Paul J. Carlson and Eun Sug Park, Texas Transportation Institute, The Texas A&M University System, College Station, Texas, and Carl K. Andersen, Office of Safety Research and Development, FHWA. Paper No. 09-0488 *The Benefits of Pavement Markings: A Renewed Perspective Based on Recent and Ongoing Research,* 2008
35. ibid
36. Rune Elvik, Alena Hoye, Truls Vaa, Michael Sorenson, Institute of Transport Economics, Oslo, Norway. *The Handbook of Road Safety Measures, Second Edition,* 2009
37. ibid

Chapter 6

1. U.S. Department of Transportation, Federal Highway Administration. *Manual on Uniform Traffic Control Devices for Streets and Highways* (MUTCD), 2009 Edition including revisions 1 and 2 dated May 2012.
2. Fig 6.6. Author: Eliot2000, Source: Own Work. Public Domain. https://commons.wikimedia.org/wiki/File:LIGHTDOME.JPG
3. Federal Highway Administration TECHNICAL ADVISORY SHOULDER AND EDGE LINE RUMBLE STRIPS T5040.39, Revision 1 November 7, 2011 and Federal Highway Administration TECHNICAL ADVISORY CENTER LINE RUMBLE STRIPS T5040.40, Revision 1 November 7, 2011
4. European Commission, Directorate General Transport. Luxembourg: Office for Official Publications of the European Communities, 1999, ISBN 92-828-6506-1. *COST 331 Requirements for Horizontal Road Marking. Final Report of the Action.*
5. U.S. Department of Transportation, Federal Highway Administration. *Manual on Uniform Traffic Control Devices for Streets and Highways* (MUTCD), 2009 Edition including revisions 1 and 2 dated May 2012.
6. AASHTO Strategic Highway Safety Plan, page 25, 2005. http://safety.transportation.org/doc/Safety-StrategicHighwaySafetyPlan.pdf

7. United States Public Law 93-87, Aug. 13, 1973, Title II, *Highway Safety Act of 1973.* http://www.gpo.gov/fdsys/pkg/STATUTE-87/pdf/STATUTE-87-Pg250.pdf

Chapter 7

1. National Highway Traffic Safety Administration (NHTSA). Traffic Safety Facts 2013
2. Federal Highway Administration (FHWA). HM-12 – Public Road Length 2013
3. Federal Highway Administration (FHWA). HM-20 – Public Road Length 2013
4. Federal Highway Administration (FHWA). VM-2 – Functional System Travel 2013
5. Federal Highway Administration (FHWA). HM-20 – Public Road Length 2013
6. National Highway Traffic Safety Administration (NHTSA). Traffic Safety Facts 2013
7. National Highway Traffic Safety Administration (NHTSA) and Federal Highway Administration (FHWA) Historical Data
8. Figure 7.1. *The Visual Link of Prevention.* Movie produced and copyrighted by Potters Industries, Inc. Written and directed by Gerald Balcar, 1982
9. Figure 7.2. *The Visual Link of Prevention.* Movie produced and copyrighted by Potters Industries, Inc. Written and directed by Gerald Balcar, 1982
10. National Highway Traffic Safety Administration (NHTSA). Traffic Safety Facts 2013
11. ibid
12. National Highway Traffic Safety Administration (NHTSA). Traffic Safety Facts 2013 and Federal Highway Administration (FHWA) Historical Data
13. National Highway Traffic Safety Administration (NHTSA). Traffic Safety Facts
14. National Highway Traffic Safety Administration (NHTSA). *Evaluation of Maine's Seat Belt Law Change From Secondary to Primary Enforcement, April, 2010.* Report No. DOT HS 811 259
15. National Highway Traffic Safety Administration (NHTSA). Traffic Safety Facts. *Seat Belt Use in 2013—Overall Results. January, 2014.* Report No. DOT HS 811 875
16. World Health Organization. *Global Status Report on Road Safety, 2015*
17. National Highway Traffic Safety Administration (NHTSA). Traffic Safety Facts
18. 1973 Highway Legislation (Highway Safety). Hearings before the Subcommittee on Transportation of the Committee on Public Works, House of Representatives, Ninety-third Congress, First Session on H.R. 2332 to Authorize Appropriations for Certain Highway Safety Projects, and for other Purposes. March 1, 6 and 7, 1973
19. ibid
20. ibid
21. IRTAD (International Road Traffic and Accident Database). Data extracted on 18 Feb, 2015
22. 1973 Highway Legislation (Highway Safety). Hearings before the Subcommittee on Transportation of the Committee on Public Works, House of Representatives, Ninety-third Congress, First Session on H.R. 2332 to Authorize Appropriations for Certain Highway Safety Projects, and for other Purposes. March 1, 6 and 7, 1973
23. ibid
24. ibid
25. Federal Highway Administration (FHWA). Highway Statistics 1973, Table DL-20, Distribution of Licensed Drivers, by Sex and Percentage in each Age Group - 1973

Chapter 8

1. World Health Organization. *Global Status Report on Road Safety,* 2015
2. IRTAD (International Road Traffic and Accident Database). Data extracted on 18 Feb, 2015. Included in high-income OECD countries are: Australia, Austria, Belgium, Canada, Denmark, Finland, France, Germany, Greece, Iceland, Ireland, Italy, Japan, Luxembourg, Netherlands, New Zealand, Norway, Portugal, Spain, Sweden, Switzerland, United Kingdom, United States
3. World Health Organization. *Global Status Report on Road Safety,* 2013
4. IRTAD (International Road Traffic and Accident Database). Data extracted on 18 Feb, 2015
5. ibid
6. World Health Organization. http://www.who.int/roadsafety/about/en/
7. World Health Organization. http://www.who.int/roadsafety/decade_of_action/friends/en/
8. World Health Organization. *World Report on Road Traffic Injury Prevention,* 2004

9. ibid
10. ibid
11. World Health Organization. *Global Status Report on Road Safety, Time for Action,* 2009
12. World Health Organization. *Global Plan for the Decade of Action for Road Safety 2011-2010.* http://www.who.int/roadsafety/decade_of_action/plan/en/
13. World Health Organization. *Global Status Report on Road Safety,* 2013
14. World Health Organization. *Global Plan for the Decade of Action for Road Safety 2011-2010.* http://www.who.int/roadsafety/decade_of_action/plan/en/
15. World Health Organization. *Global Status Report on Road Safety,* 2013
16. ibid
17. ibid
18. Meeting Report from "Meeting of the friends of the decade of action for road safety 2011-2020. 14 November 2014, Brasilia, Brazil"
19. United Nations Economic Commission for Europe (UNECE). http://www.unece.org/un-sgs-special-envoy-for-road-safety/un-sgs-special-envoy-for-road-safety.html
20. FIA (Fédération Internationale de l'Automobile). http://www.fia.com/organisation
21. The FIA Foundation. http://www.fiafoundation.org/about-us
22. United Nations Economic Commission for Europe (UNECE). http://www.unece.org/un-sgs-special-envoy-for-road-safety/un-sgs-special-envoy-for-road-safety.html
23. United Nations. http://www.un.org/sustainabledevelopment/sustainable-development-goals/
24. World Health Organization. *Global Status Report on Road Safety,* 2015
25. ibid
26. World Health Organization. *Global Status Report on Road Safety,* 2015 – Summary
27. Brasilia Declaration on Road Safety. November, 2015. http://www.who.int/violence_injury_prevention/road_traffic/Brasilia_Declaration/en/
28. World Health Organization. http://www.who.int/violence_injury_prevention/road_traffic/Zero_draft_of_the_Brasilia_Declaration_on_Road_Safety_26_March_2015_FINAL.pdf?ua=1
29. World Health Organization. http://www.who.int/violence_injury_prevention/road_traffic/Final_Brasilia_declaration_EN.pdf?ua=1
30. The FIA Foundation. http://www.fiafoundation.org/blog/2015/november/brasilia-declaration-sets-manifesto-for-change-to-meet-global-goals
31. Norman L.G. *Road traffic accidents: epidemiology, control, and prevention.* World Health Organization, Geneva, 1962.
32. World Health Organization. *World Report on Road Traffic Injury Prevention,* 2004
33. Federal Highway Administration (FHWA). Persons Fatally Injured in Motor Vehicle Crashes 1967-1995. April 1997. Table FI-210
34. World Health Organization. *Global Status Report on Road Safety,* 2015

Conclusion

1. European Commission, Directorate General Transport. Luxembourg: Office for Official Publications of the European Communities, 1999, ISBN 92-828-6506-1. *COST 331 Requirements for Horizontal Road Marking. Final Report of the Action.*
2. Rune Elvik, Alena Hoye, Truls Vaa, Michael Sorenson, Institute of Transport Economics, Oslo, Norway. *The Handbook of Road Safety Measures, Second Edition,* 2009
3. World Health Organization. *Global Plan for the Decade of Action for Road Safety 2011-2010.* http://www.who.int/roadsafety/decade_of_action/plan/en/
4. World Health Organization. *Global Status Report on Road Safety,* 2015

Glossary

Arterial Roads, Minor: Mostly two-lane roads between rural or small urban centers or from such centers to Limited Access Highways. They may connect housing developments to rural or urban centers.

Arterial Roads, Principal: Roads between urban population or business centers or from such centers to Limited Access Highways. Can be multi-lane or two-lane.

Balanced Approach: The concept promoted in the Highway Safety Act of 1966 of approximate equal funding and attention to all different behavior modification efforts to reduce crashes, and to efforts for surviving crashes, ranging in activities from driver education programs to emergency medical services. Safety improvements to roads to mitigate the number of crashes resulting from driver mistakes was not specifically included. This "balanced approach" fails to use priorities of action.

Center Lines: On two-lane roads, double solid lines indicate no incursion over the lines and dashed line patterns indicate safe passing zones or safe incursion into the opposite direction traffic lane if no opposite direction vehicles are in sight or are at a safe distance. Where the lines are yellow, they indicate opposite direction traffic on the other side of the line. On four-lane roads where they are used, double solid lines indicate no incursion in the opposite direction lanes. If the lines are white, a double solid line indicates opposite direction traffic on the opposite side with incursion or passing zones indicated with dashed line patterns on two-lane roads.

Collector Roads, Major: Multi-lane or two-lane roads gathering traffic from local or residential roads to convey to rural or urban centers or to Arterial Roads.

Collector Roads, Minor: Two-lane roads that gather residential traffic in suburbs or in rural areas to take it to various centers or to Arterial Roads.

Controlled Access Highway: See Limited Access Highway

Edge Lines: On two-lane roads, these are almost universally white solid lines along the pavement edge indicating shoulder paving or soft turf opposite the line. Some uses show broken edge lines alongside passing zones on wide two-lane roads where slower traffic can move to a parallel lane or shoulder lane to allow same direction passing. On roads with more than two lanes, edge lines are nearly universal in rich world nations.

Expressway: A Limited Access Highway, usually in an urban area.

Federal-Aid Roads: An earlier American system of rural and urban Arterial and Collector Roads, or primary and secondary roads, eligible for programs partially or fully paid for by federally appropriated funds.

Federal Highway Administration (FHWA): A United States agency, under the Department of Transportation, which was originally the Bureau of Public Roads from 1905. It sets standards and plans for the American road infrastructure and issues funds and monitors actions for new road and bridge construction, repair and maintenance. It sets standards for American roads, including road safety as the road infrastructure is concerned. It is responsible for all road travel and related data.

Foveal Vision: Also called "central vision," is that approximately 7% of the total visual field of the human eye used for reading and scrutinizing. The balance is "peripheral vision" where objects and actions are detected to serve as a spatial guide to walking or driving and for warnings.

Glass Beads: Glass beads are the retroreflective element in pavement markings. They are made from lead free, recycled soda lime glass. The original industrial application for such beads in Renaissance Europe was for grinding pigments for dyes and paints. These beads were produced in small carbon matrix furnaces. Rudolph and Paul Potters, sales representatives of German producers, established a factory in Brooklyn, NY in 1914 when imports from Germany were interrupted at the outbreak of World War I. When in the early 1920s, new demand for coating motion picture screens with glass beads required larger and cheaper production capabilities, the Potters brothers developed a vertical furnace technology that produced glass beads in an upward flowing stream of super-heated gasses. The company, which became Potters Industries, is the world leader in this technology, now many generations improved. In addition to its use in pavement markings, glass beads are used for blast cleaning and shot peening metals, for medical applications in burn treatment and for coating for incorporation in electronic shielding and conductive materials.

Highway Safety Act of 1966: Faced by increases in fatalities on America's roads, the House of Representatives Committee on Public Works, led by chairman George Fallon, put together what they thought was a grand design of a highway safety bill with a "balanced approach." It established standards for road safety and was signed into law September 9, 1966. By 1971, road traffic fatalities were still increasing.

Highway Safety Act of 1973: Formed in the House Committee on Public Works beginning in 1971 as HR-2332, instigated and sponsored by William Harsha, Ranking Republican, it was cosponsored by every member of the committee. It was passed by the Senate on the consent calendar as S-893. The House of Representatives then merged it into The Federal Aid Highway Act of 1973 as Title 2, which was signed into law August 12, 1973.

Highway Trust Fund: The American repository for gasoline taxes, now 18.4 cents per gallon, for funding road construction, repair, expansion and road safety.

Interstate Highway System: A national network of Limited Access Highways in the United States. As of 2013, about 25% of American road traffic is on this system.

Limited Access Highway: Generally, four-lane or wider roads with a median divider between opposite direction lanes. Access is controlled or limited to entrance ramps with a lane merge and no intersections, stop signs or traffic controls. Exiting is by an exit lane and egress ramp. Known as "motorways" in the UK.

MADD (Mothers Against Drunk Driving): A national US organization formed by Candace Lightner after her daughter was killed by a drunk driver. It was accorded success in changing American culture to emphasize efforts to mitigate impaired driving.

National Highway Traffic Safety Administration (NHTSA): The agency created in the United States, under the Department of Transportation, that emerged from the reorganization of the National Highway Safety Bureau that was created by the National Traffic and Motor Vehicle Safety Act of 1966. It is intended to fund and administer the programs established by the act but with action programs carried out by the states. It is responsible for research grants. It also issues and monitors federal vehicle safety standards. Further, NHTSA sees to the collection and publishing of road traffic crash data.

National Traffic and Motor Vehicle Safety Act of 1966: Companion legislation to the Highway Safety Act of 1966 focused on the first national vehicle safety standards in the United States. It established a new agency to oversee the standards that later became the National Highway Traffic Safety Agency (NHTSA) in 1970. It was signed into law the same day as the Highway Safety Act of 1966, September 9, 1966.

OECD: The Organisation for Economic Co-operation and Development.

Parkways: Limited Access Highways reserved for passenger cars and light vehicles.

Passing Zones: Areas of tested sight distance on two-lane roads where cars travelling at the speed limit can pass slower vehicles travelling in the same direction if no opposite direction vehicles are seen or are a sufficient distance away.

Pavement Marking: The application of specialized paint, thermo-plastic and other materials to road pavements as center lines, edge lines and various other markings. A glass bead refractive index of 1.5 is used for horizontal retroreflectivity. Beads may be dropped on at application and/or premixed into the binder.

Pavement Marking Demonstration Program: The road safety action program for road marking included in the Highway Safety Act of 1973. Federal funding of 100% of expenditures was made available to the states to center-line and edge-line marking of rural roads.

The idea was to let them find out if pavement markings were indeed an effective crash countermeasure.

Peripheral Vision: The more than 90% of the visual field of the human eye that positions persons by seeing and sensing guide factors. This is the vision and brain interlock on edge lines during driving.

Population Fatality Rate or Population Death Rate: Road traffic fatalities per 100,000 population.

Presidential Commission on Drunk Driving: Established in April 1982 by Executive Order 12358 signed by President Ronald Reagan with 26 members and one year to produce a final report. This focused on stronger enforcement but included a recommendation for center lines and edge lines.

Random Breath Testing: Generally a European practice of stopping drivers for a random breath check for blood alcohol level with no indication of violation.

Reflectorized vs. Retroreflectorized: These generally mean the same retroreflection of head light beams. See Retroreflectivity.

Retroreflectivity: The capacity of glass beaded horizontal paint or plastic road pavement markings, or beaded vertical signs or prismatic reflectors, to directly return the light from vehicle headlights at night. All signs and markings are retroreflective. The term "reflectorized" markings or signs used herein is a contraction whereas the correct, but more cumbersome, word is "retroreflectorized."

Road Marking: See Pavement Marking.

Road Safety Engineering: Improving the safety of the existing road infrastructure, primarily by installing and maintaining reflectorized center lines with passing zones and edge lines, upgrading intersections, removing obstacles and upgrading rail crossings.

Toll Road: A Limited Access Highway funded by government authorities or private investment for which tolls are collected from users to pay for the construction and maintenance thereof. The French Autoroutes and the Italian Autostrade are examples. Some US highways like the New York State Thruway and the Pennsylvania Turnpike are also toll roads.

Two-lane Road: Roads with two traffic lanes with traffic in opposite directions with no median divider. Known as "single carriageways" in the UK.

US House of Representatives: That part of the US Congress with 435 members representing the 50 states according to population. The US Senate has two senators from each state, totaling 100 members. Both units of congress must agree on all bills sent to the president for approval. Each has standing committees looking after areas of legislation. These committees become institutions. The House Committee on Transportation and Infrastructure, formerly The Committee on Public Works, originates all funding bills for roads of all types, road safety, railroads and airports. Twenty-six states are represented on this committee.

Index

A

AAA 103. *See also* American Automobile Association
AASHO 14. *See also* American Association of State Highway Officials
AASHTO 103, 161. *See also* American Association of State Highway and Transportation Officials
ADT 41, 98, 102, 103. *See also* average daily traffic
alcohol impaired driving 56, 68
Allen, Merrill 65–68
American Association of Motor Vehicle Administrators 122
American Association of State Highway Officials 14. *See also* AASHO
American Association of State Highway and Transportation Officials 103, 161. *See also* AASHTO
American Automobile Association 14, 103. *See also* AAA
American Road and Transportation Builders Association 14, 107. *See also* ARTBA
Anderson, Carl 86
ARTBA 14, 107. *See also* American Road and Transportation Builders Association
Austria 5, 51, 52, 63, 129, 162
average daily traffic 20, 36, 41, 84, 98. *See also* ADT

B

BAC 57, 58, 62, 63, 71–73, 76–78, 115, 117, 142, 159, 160. *See also* blood alcohol content
BBC 57, 59
bicycle lanes 56, 64, 141
Blatnik, John 35, 47, 48
blood alcohol content 57, 71, 117. *See also* BAC
Bloomberg Philanthropies 131, 133
Brasilia Declaration 135, 136, 163
Breslin, James 50, 70
Bretton-Woods Agreement of 1944 51
British road studs 94

C

Canada 5, 6, 60, 62, 63, 83, 95, 129, 160, 162
Carlson, Paul 85, 161
center lines 2, 6, 8, 12–15, 17–20, 22–26, 39–41, 45, 47, 48, 52–55, 65–69, 74, 86–90, 96–103, 105, 107, 112, 113, 118, 12–123, 137, 140, 141, 147–149, 168, 169

child restraints 132, 134, 139, 142
China 5
Committee on Public Works (US House of Representatives) 1, 31, 34, 35, 38, 44, 47, 48, 70, 119, 158, 159, 162, 167, 170, 176, 177
Committee on the Environment and Public Works (US Senate) 31
Committee on Transportation and Infrastructure (US House of Representative) 37, 170
Connor, Robert E. (Bob) 16, 49, 50
COST 331 9, 55, 79, 80–82, 99, 148, 159, 161, 163
countermeasure 6, 25, 69, 81–83, 85, 89, 98, 103, 105, 107, 116, 120, 147, 148, 150, 168
crosswalks 1, 104, 120, 147

D

daylight running lights 66
DeLade, Charles 49
Department of Transportation 16, 32, 101, 102, 157, 161, 166, 168
developing world 1, 3, 8, 9, 123, 149, 150–154
DUI 56, 57, 58, 62, 159, 160. *See also* driving under the influence
driving under the influence 57, 62, 110, 142. *See also* DUI
Dykstra, James 50, 70

E

edge lines 2, 6, 8, 15–23, 25, 26, 39, 40–42, 45, 47, 48, 52–55, 65, 66–71, 74–78, 82, 83, 85–89, 96, 97, 100, 102–105, 107, 112, 113, 118, 120–123, 137, 140, 141, 147–149, 166, 168, 169
EEA 60. *See also* European Economic Area
Enfield, Clifford (Cliff) 34, 49
epoxy 16, 37, 92, 97, 99, 172
Ethiopia 5, 126
European Commission 9, 55, 79, 80, 99, 148, 159, 161, 163
European Economic Area 60. *See also* EEA
European Union 55, 56, 60, 61, 79, 80

F

Fallon, George 32, 167
fatal crashes 20, 23–25, 103, 140
fatality rates 5, 57, 61, 63, 64, 127–129, 154
Federal Aid Highway Act of 1956 28
Federal Aid Highway Act of 1973 107, 119, 120, 167
Federal Aid Highway System 31, 107
Federal Highway Administration 1, 16, 31, 34, 38, 44, 47, 49, 50, 54, 69, 78, 99, 101, 117, 119, 129, 157–159, 161, 162, 163, 166. *See also* FHWA

FHWA 16, 17, 31, 37, 46, 78, 84, 86, 101, 102, 117, 119, 120, 129, 138, 157–159, 161–163, 166. *See also* Federal Highway Administration
FIA (Fédération Internationale de l'Automobile) 134, 163
FIA Foundation 134, 136, 163
first responder network 142
France 5, 7, 51, 52, 56, 58, 59, 62, 63, 128, 129, 159, 162
Friends of the Decade 130. *See also* Friends of the Decade of Action for Road Safety 2011-2020
Friends of the Decade of Action for Road Safety 2011-2020 130. *See also* Friends of the Decade

G

Gates, Timothy J. 83, 161
Germany 8, 5, 7, 19, 20, 52, 53, 58–60, 63, 128, 129, 162, 166
glass beads 15, 16, 35, 36, 54, 90–92, 96, 97, 99, 101, 166, 167
Global Ministerial Conference on Road Safety 8, 131
Global Plan for the Decade of Action for Road Safety 2011-2020 8, 130–133, 136, 139, 140, 143, 144, 149, 150, 157. *See also* WHO Global Plan
Global Status Report on Road Safety 2013, Supporting a Decade of Action 133
Global Status Report on Road Safety 2015 126–128, 135, 149, 154
Global Status Report on Road Safety, Time for Action 131, 163
Governor's Highway Safety Representatives 118, 119
guardrails 113

H

Haddon, Jr., Dr. William 29, 30, 34, 137,148
Haddon Matrix 30
Handbook of Road Safety Measures 86, 161, 163
Harsha, William (Bill) 35, 39, 44, 47, 48, 50, 119–121, 149, 167
Hawkins, H. Gene 83, 161
headlights 66, 81, 90, 98, 169
head-on collisions 22, 25
helmets 56, 132, 134, 139, 142, 143
Highway Safety Act of 1966 8, 31, 33, 34, 38, 46, 52, 112, 118, 158, 165, 167, 168
Highway Safety Act of 1973 8, 37, 41–44, 47, 48, 52, 107, 112, 118–120, 158, 162, 167, 168
Highway Trust Fund 14, 28, 43, 44, 107, 120, 167
House of Representatives 1, 31, 32, 34, 35, 38, 48, 158, 159, 162, 167, 170
Howard, James 49

I

IIHS 29, 158. *See also* Insurance Institute for Highway Safety
IMF 51, 126–128, 144. *See also* International Monetary Fund

impaired driving 32, 48, 56, 57, 62, 68, 114, 115, 117, 123, 142, 168
India 5, 126, 144, 155
Indonesia 5, 126
Institute of Traffic Engineers 16
Institute of Transport Economics 9, 86, 148, 161, 163
Insurance Institute for Highway Safety 29. *See also* IIHS
International Monetary Fund 51, 157. *See also* IMF
International Road Federation 145
Interstate and Defense Highway System 14, 28, 31, 53, 107, 167
Iran 5, 126, 127
Italy 5, 7, 51, 52, 58, 62, 63, 129, 162

J

Japan 2, 5, 6, 7, 49, 60, 63, 128, 129, 140, 162, 171
Johnson, Lyndon 29, 32

K

Kreml, Franklin 119, 121

L

Lamm, Lester 47, 49
Lightner, Candace 46, 114, 167
limited access highway 166, 167, 169
livable cities 64
low- and middle-income countries 2, 5, 6, 9, 52, 82, 87, 105, 125, 129, 132, 133, 135, 139, 143–146, 148, 153, 154

M

MADD 46, 114, 115, 167. *See also* Mothers Against Drunk Driving
McCarroll, June 12, 13, 158
Magnuson, Warren G. 34
Mandela, Zoleka 136
Manley, John 37, 49
Manual and Specifications for the Manufacture, Display, and Erection of U.S. Standard Road Markers and Signs 14
Manual on Street Traffic Signs, Signals and Markings 14
Manual on Uniform Traffic Control Devices 14, 89, 101, 161. *See also* MUTCD
Marshall Plan, The 51
May, Walter R. 35, 48, 120
Mothers Against Drunk Driving 46, 47, 69, 114, 167. *See also* MADD
Motor Vehicle Manufacturers Association 119. *See also* MVMA
MUTCD 14–17, 89, 101–104, 161. *See also* Manual on Uniform Traffic Control Devices

MVMA 119, 121. *See also* Motor Vehicle Manufacturers Association

N

Nader, Ralph 30, 111, 148
National Action Committee for Highway Safety 27
National Conference on Street and Highway Safety 14. *See also* NCSHS
National Highway Traffic Safety Administration 29, 115, 157–160, 162, 168. *See also* NHTSA
National Safety Council 31, 33, 121
National Traffic and Motor Vehicle Safety Act of 1966 8, 33, 168
National Traffic Safety Agency 29, 30
NCSHS 14. *See also* National Conference on Street and Highway Safety
NHTSA 29, 31, 115, 116, 157–160, 162, 168. *See also* National Highway Traffic Safety Administration
Nigeria 5, 126
night driving 37, 66
Norway 51, 60, 62–64, 86, 128, 148, 161–163
Norwegian Ministry of Transportation and Communication 86
Norwegian Public Roads Administration 86

O

OECD (Organisation for Economic Co-operation and Development) 1, 5, 63, 125, 159, 162
O'Leary, Timothy H. (Tim) 49

P

Pakistan 5, 126
Park, Dr. Eun Sug 86
pavement marking 2, 6, 11, 35–39, 42, 44, 52–55, 65, 70, 79, 80, 85, 90, 105, 107, 108, 113, 116, 120, 121
Pavement Marking Demonstration Program 9, 41, 47, 86, 168
pedestrian islands 120
Peet, Richard C. (Dick) 35, 48, 50, 120
perfected road system 64, 147
peripheral vision 66, 67, 166, 169
Potters Industries 16, 35, 37, 38, 49, 68, 69, 74, 91, 92, 101, 158–160, 162, 167
Presidential Commission on Drunk Driving 46, 47, 69, 114, 169
President's Committee on Traffic Safety 33

R

raised pavement markers 94–97
reflectorized lines 2, 6, 8, 36, 39, 40, 45, 48, 52, 53, 67, 69, 79, 89, 96, 97, 104, 107, 112, 113, 120, 123, 137, 141, 147–149, 169

retroreflectivity 15, 54, 55, 69, 81–83, 85, 90, 92, 96, 98–100, 168
rich world 1, 2, 5, 7–9, 34, 89, 104, 108, 114, 117, 131, 133, 137, 147, 148, 150, 151, 152, 154, 166, 171
risk factors 8, 130, 133–135, 139
Ritter, James R. (Jim) 49, 74
Rivard, Lloyd 35, 48, 120
road delineation 13, 27
road marking 17, 18, 20, 25, 26, 35, 39, 50, 55, 65, 80–83, 87, 90, 101, 103, 148, 168
road safety engineering 2, 6, 7, 8, 39, 42, 44, 47, 50, 52, 53, 55, 59, 64, 89, 112–114, 117–121, 123, 129, 137, 139, 141, 143, 147–152, 154
road safety programs 32, 53, 119, 121, 122, 123, 141
road traffic fatalities 1, 3, 5, 8, 9, 28, 34, 39, 48, 52, 111, 112, 116, 122, 125, 133, 135, 136, 143, 151, 154, 155, 167
Roe, Robert A. 35, 37, 49, 50
Rutgers Center for Alcohol Studies 71, 72

S

safe system 55, 64, 113, 114, 138, 147
seatbelts 6, 34, 56, 59, 60, 116, 117, 121, 134, 137, 139, 142, 143, 148
seatbelt use 46–48, 56, 58, 59, 64, 110, 113, 114, 116, 141
Second Global High-Level Conference on Road Safety 135
Senate 1, 30–33, 37, 119, 167, 170
Senate Commerce Committee 1, 30, 33
Shuster, E. G. (Bud) 49
specialized lanes 104
speed 11, 45, 46, 59, 81, 86, 91, 110, 117, 132, 133, 139, 141, 168, 171
Subcommittee on Investigations and Oversight (US House of Representatives) 37, 48, 70
Subcommittee on Transportation of the Committee on Public Works (US House of Representatives) 38, 158, 159, 162
Sullivan, Richard 35, 48, 120
Sustainable Development Goals 128, 134, 135
Sweden 5, 7, 51, 52, 57, 58, 60, 62–64, 128, 129, 162

T

Texas Transportation Institute 82, 86, 161, 176
Thailand 5, 126, 127
thermoplastic 16, 37, 54, 92, 93, 97, 99
Todt, Jean 134
traffic laws 8, 27, 61, 114, 129, 138, 141
traffic safety data 142
Transportation Research Record 78, 160, 161
Truman, Harry 27

tunnel vision 67
two-wheeled 105, 126, 141, 142, 143, 154

U

United Kingdom 5, 7, 52, 57, 60, 62–64, 94, 128, 129, 162
United Nations 9, 1, 2, 8, 51, 129, 130, 132, 163. *See also* UN
United Nations Road Safety Collaboration 130. *See also* UNRSC
United States 5, 6, 7, 11, 14, 16, 20, 26–28, 31, 34, 42, 45, 47, 50–55, 57–63, 69, 80, 81, 83, 86–89, 95, 99, 101–103, 107, 109, 110, 112–115, 120–122, 127, 129, 138, 140, 147, 149, 157, 158, 162, 166–168, 171
UN 2, 3, 8, 9, 130, 134–137, 145, 146, 151–153,179. *See also* United Nations
UNRSC 130, 131. *See also* United Nations Road Safety Collaboration
UN/WHO 9, 2, 3, 8, 135, 137, 151, 152. *See also* UN

V

vehicle safety standards 1, 110, 147, 149, 151, 153, 154, 168
Vision Zero 8, 48, 55, 64, 113, 147

W

Wagner, Jason 85, 161
walking 27, 59, 64, 66, 67, 90, 104, 111, 112, 117, 143, 166
Way, John 50, 70
Western Europe 2, 6, 17, 20, 31, 48, 51–57, 59–62, 64, 65, 69, 81, 82, 99, 110, 111, 113, 116, 120, 121, 140, 147, 171
white center line 12, 41, 102
WHO 2, 3, 8, 9, 60,126–128, 130–139, 143, 145, 146, 150–155, 179. *See also* World Health Organization
WHO Global Plan 8, 139, 143, 150. *See also* Global Plan for the Decade of Action for Road Safety 2011-2020
WHO Report 2004 9. *See also* World Report on Road Traffic Injury Prevention
WHO Report 2009 135. *See also* Global Status Report on Road Safety, Time for Action
WHO Report 2013 135. *See also* Global Status Report on Road Safety 2013
Wood, Thomas K. 49
World Health Organization 1, 2, 8, 130, 149, 157, 159–163. *See also* WHO
World Report on Road Traffic Injury Prevention 8, 9, 130, 138 157, 162, 163
World War II 15, 19, 27, 48, 51, 94

Y

yellow center line 11, 12, 17, 36, 55

About the Authors

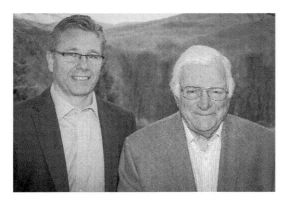

Bo and Gerry at company HQ in Margaretville in the Catskill Mountains upstate New York.

Gerry Balcar was one of a small group called upon by a US congressional committee in the early 1970s to determine whether making existing roads safer would have the effect of preventing road traffic crashes. Government officials had been unable to stem an unprecedented increase in such crashes and subsequent fatalities in the United States that had begun in the early 1960s. Tighter laws, more enforcement and appeals to obey speed limits, to abstain from drinking and driving, and other behavior modification countermeasures had not worked.

For more than ten years, Gerry was involved in refocusing road traffic safety efforts to improving existing roads in the rich world. He gave lectures, provided testimony and conducted new research in the US and participated in related meetings in Western Europe and Japan. No one of those involved at the time realized they were inaugurating a historic change in road safety thinking.

Bo Elfving has been deeply engaged in this change and has proposed recommendations of doable solutions that developing countries can implement quickly. Bo brings an up-to-date perspective to the research for this book as well as to its writing.

Made in the USA
San Bernardino, CA
24 February 2017